Breast Cancer Treatment by Focused Microwave Thermotherapy

Alan J. Fenn, PhD
Massachusetts Institute of Technology
Cambridge, Massachusetts

JONES AND BARTLETT PUBLISHERS

Sudbury, Massachusetts

BOSTON   TORONTO   LONDON   SINGAPORE

World Headquarters
Jones and Bartlett Publishers
40 Tall Pine Drive
Sudbury, MA 01776
978-443-5000
info@jbpub.com
www.jbpub.com

Jones and Bartlett Publishers
Canada
6339 Ormindale Way
Mississauga, Ontario L5V 1J2
CANADA

Jones and Bartlett Publishers
International
Barb House, Barb Mews
London W6 7PA
UK

Jones and Bartlett's books and products are available through most bookstores and online booksellers. To contact Jones and Bartlett Publishers directly, call 800-832-0034, fax 978-443-8000, or visit our website, www.jbpub.com.

Substantial discounts on bulk quantities of Jones and Bartlett's publications are available to corporations, professional associations, and other qualified organizations. For details and specific discount information, contact the special sales department at Jones and Bartlett via the above contact information or send an email to specialsales@jbpub.com.

The authors, editor, and publisher have made every effort to provide accurate information. However, they are not responsible for errors, omissions, or for any outcomes related to the use of the contents of this book and take no responsibility for the use of the products described. Treatments and side effects described in this book may not be applicable to all patients; likewise, some patients may require a dose or experience a side effect that is not described herein. The reader should confer with his or her own physician regarding specific treatments and side effects. Drugs and medical devices are discussed that may have limited availability controlled by the Food and Drug Administration (FDA) for use only in a research study or clinical trial. The drug information presented has been derived from reference sources, recently published data, and pharmaceutical research data. Research, clinical practice, and government regulations often change the accepted standard in this field. When consideration is being given to use of any drug in the clinical setting, the healthcare provider or reader is responsible for determining FDA status of the drug, reading the package insert, reviewing prescribing information for the most up-to-date recommendations on dose, precautions, and contraindications, and determining the appropriate usage for the product. This is especially important in the case of drugs that are new or seldom used.

Library of Congress Cataloging-in-Publication Data
Fenn, A. J. (Alan Jeffrey), 1953-
  Breast cancer treatment by focused microwave thermotherapy /
Alan J. Fenn.
    p. ; cm.
  Includes bibliographical references and index.
  ISBN-13: 978-0-7637-4870-8 (alk. paper)
  ISBN-10: 0-7637-4870-6 (alk. paper)
  1. Breast--Cancer--Thermotherapy.   I. Title.
  [DNLM: 1. Breast Neoplasms--therapy. 2. Hyperthermia, Induced
--methods. 3. Microwaves--therapeutic use.   WP 870 F334b 2007]
  RC280.B8F456 2007
  616.99'44906--dc22

                                        2006024456

WP
870
F334b
2007

6048

Production Credits

Executive Publisher: Christopher Davis
Production Director: Amy Rose
Associate Editor: Kathy Richardson
Production Assistant: Amanda Clerkin
Associate Marketing Manager: Laura Kavigian
Composition: Jason Miranda, Spoke & Wheel

V.P., Manufacturing and Inventory Control:
  Therese Connell
Cover Design: Jan Van Aarsen
Cover Image: © Brand X Pictures/Alamy Images
Printing and Binding: Malloy, Inc.
Cover Printing: Malloy, Inc

Printed in the United States of America
10 09 08 07 06   10 9 8 7 6 5 4 3 2 1

To My Family

Contents

Preface

The development of new treatment modalities for improving the clinical outcomes for patients with breast cancer is a major challenge. For example, current standard-of-care breast conservation treatment of invasive breast cancer often involves a wide-excision lumpectomy (partial mastectomy) to remove the primary tumor and a surrounding wide margin of tissue, followed by radiation therapy to destroy any residual tumor cells in the breast. Although standard breast conservation surgery generally is very effective, in some cases viable tumor cells remain at the surgical margins after wide excision and, if not reexcised, even with postoperative radiation therapy, these residual cancer cells can lead to an increased risk for a local recurrence of the cancer. Furthermore, breast conservation currently is underutilized, and physicians and patients often select a mastectomy approach for treatment, in some cases because patients prefer not to undergo postoperative radiation therapy, which can involve numerous, time-consuming, fractionated treatments and has many side effects. It is desirable to consider new adjuvant treatment modalities that are noninvasive or minimally invasive that could lead to a more complete elimination of viable breast cancer cells without added side effects, and that improve the overall effectiveness of breast conservation. In the future, if all cancer cells in the breast can be completely and reliably destroyed by a new treatment modality alone, or in combination with other treatment modalities, it might be possible to eliminate or reduce breast surgery and/or radiation therapy and potentially increase the utilization and effectiveness of breast conservation.

A new breast cancer treatment modality currently under investigation in clinical research by a number of groups is referred to as *thermotherapy*, which is applied by various types of energy sources to the breast using thermal effects to ablate cancer cells. One particular breast thermotherapy method being explored involves externally focused microwave energy to elevate, hypothetically, the temperature of the primary breast cancer tumor and cancer cells in the margins to a sufficient temperature and for a period of heating that will ablate all the visible and microscopic cancer cells. Breast cancer cells generally have higher water content and higher ion content compared to the surrounding normal breast tissues such as fat, glandular, ductal, and connective tissues. Microwaves are known to selectively target high-water-content/high-ion-content tissues, which could allow for preferential heating of cancerous breast tumors as well as precancerous and noncancerous breast lesions. Additional selective heating of tumor cells can be achieved by focusing the microwave energy on the breast tumor region with two or more coherent applicators (a phased array of transmitting antennas) surrounding the breast. Focused microwave thermotherapy delivered transcutaneously to malignant breast tumors and to the surrounding margins could provide a means for completely sterilizing the tumor region using heat alone prior to surgery. The transcutaneous antenna array, with electric-field feedback from a minimally invasive microwave probe positioned (under ultrasound guidance) in the tumor mass, and an adaptive phased array control system can be used in supplying a focused microwave field for heating breast tumors in the compressed breast.

Recently, preoperative focused microwave phased array breast thermotherapy, typically administered in one or two treatments, has been investigated in clinical studies and has shown promising results for patients with invasive breast cancer. Clinical studies of heat-alone focused microwave thermotherapy prior to surgery (partial mastectomy or mastectomy) for patients with small to large breast carcinomas have been conducted. For patients with large breast cancer tumors, a study of preoperative focused microwave thermotherapy used in combination with preoperative chemotherapy has also been conducted.

The objective of this book is to review for medical students; surgical, medical, and radiation oncologists; pathologists; medical physicists; biomedical and electrical engineers; other specialists; and breast cancer researchers the clinical rationale, theory, technology, methods, and preclinical and clinical results for breast cancer treatment by ultrasound-guided focused microwave phased array thermotherapy. The generation of focused microwaves and the theory and analysis for preferential heating of cancerous and benign breast lesions in normal breast tissue by microwave energy are described in detail. The results of preclinical phantom and animal testing for focused microwave phased array thermotherapy are reviewed. In Phase I and Phase II clinical studies for breast cancer patients, focused microwave phased array thermotherapy is shown to kill breast cancer cells and induce tumor shrinkage. The results of a randomized clinical study suggest that preoperative transcutaneous focused microwave thermotherapy can induce tumor cell necrosis and might reduce the rate of positive margins for patients with invasive breast cancer who receive breast-conserving surgery. The results of a randomized study of preoperative focused microwave thermotherapy in combination with preoperative chemotherapy for patients with large breast cancer tumors are also reviewed, and the results suggest an increase in tumor shrinkage with thermochemotherapy compared to chemotherapy alone. Based on the data reviewed in this monograph, future applications and clinical rationale are outlined, including the treatment of small and large breast cancer tumors in the intact breast, recurrent chest wall breast cancer, precancerous ductal carcinoma in situ, breast cancer prevention, and treatment of benign breast conditions.

The data contained in this monograph are results of the efforts of a number of colleagues, most notably for the clinical results: Dr. Hernan I. Vargas, Dr. William C. Dooley, Dr. Robert A. Gardner, Dr. Sylvia Heywang-Köbrunner, Dr. Mary Beth Tomaselli, Dr. Jay K. Harness, Dr. Christine T. Mroz, Dr. Lynne P. Clark, Dr. Claire M. Carman, Dr. Sandra B. Schultz, Dr. John Winstanley, Dr. Gary V. Kuehl, Dr. Mariana Doval, and Dr. Jerome B. Block. Other significant support and encouragement for development and demonstration of the adaptive phased array focused microwave thermotherapy technology for breast cancer came from, most notably for early preclinical development, Mr. Donald H. Temme, Mr. James Fitzgerald, and Mr. Robert J. Burns; for technology transfer, Ms. Lori Pressman; for animal studies, Dr. Jeffrey W. Hand; and for development of the clinical breast thermotherapy system, Dr. Augustine Y. Cheung, Mr. John Mon, and Mr. Dennis Smith.

Clinical Rationale for Focused Microwave Thermotherapy for Invasive Breast Cancer

Thermotherapy for Invasive Breast Cancer

1.1 INTRODUCTION

The treatment of breast cancer has evolved considerably in the last few decades as a result, in part, of changes in clinical presentation as described by Edney.[1] Improved and increased patient education and awareness, public support, and improved and increased use of screening mammography have contributed to a decrease in the size of detected breast cancer as described by Cady.[2] Patients with operable breast cancer are treated by breast-conserving surgery (BCS) referred to as *partial mastectomy* (with or without axillary lymph node dissection) or by mastectomy (with or without axillary lymph node dissection).

For improved breast conservation, less invasive and improved diagnostic and treatment procedures have been developed. These improved procedures include biopsy methodology such as core needle or vacuum-assisted biopsy instead of excisional biopsy, wide-excision lumpectomy or partial mastectomy instead of mastectomy, multicolor inking (instead of single-color inking) at the cut edges of the resection specimen to identify the orientation of margins along with improved understanding of the impact of pathologic tumor margins, sentinel lymph node mapping and biopsy instead of complete axillary lymph node dissection, whole breast and partial breast radiation therapy to follow BCS to reduce local recurrence, preoperative chemotherapy for reducing the size of large tumors to enable breast conservation, and more recently breast tumor ablation prior to surgery. Each type of procedure has been increasingly explored in clinical practice and in clinical research for the treatment of breast cancer.[3-6]

In the case of breast conservation (lumpectomy) compared to mastectomy, with 20-year follow-up from the National Surgical Adjuvant Breast and Bowel Project (NSABP) B-6, patients that received breast conservation treatment (lumpectomy plus radiation therapy) had an equivalent survival rate (approximately 50% in each of three arms—lumpectomy, lumpectomy and radiation, and mastectomy) compared to those patients that received a mastectomy as described by Fisher et al.[3] In NSABP B-6, patients that received lumpectomy alone had a local recurrence rate of 39.2%, whereas patients receiving lumpectomy plus radiation therapy had a local recurrence rate of only 14.3%—radiation therapy is currently an important component of breast conservation to eliminate residual cancer cells not excised by surgery and to reduce recurrence.

The goals of any improved breast conservation procedure are to conserve as much breast tissue as possible for cosmetic purposes while achieving negative margins for invasive and *in situ* carcinomas and to reduce breast cancer recurrence rates without significant added side effects. Section 1.2 describes a recent breast cancer treatment modality using preoperative transcutaneous (externally applied through the skin) focused microwave thermotherapy (FMT) to ablate (kill) carcinoma cells prior to BCS. Section 1.3 discusses the importance of preventing close or positive surgical margins for tumor cells in breast conservation treatments, and Section 1.4 reviews the current utilization rates for standard breast conservation and mastectomy procedures. Section 1.5 discusses a novel approach for using preoperative FMT in combination with preoperative chemotherapy for reducing the size of large breast carcinomas to improve surgical options and to allow breast conservation instead of mastectomy.

1.2 BREAST CANCER TUMOR ABLATION USING FOCUSED MICROWAVE PHASED ARRAY THERMOTHERAPY

Breast cancer tumor ablation by thermotherapy as part of a multi-modality approach in the treatment of breast cancer has been the subject of a number of recent studies.[4-6] Tumor ablation methods for treatment of breast cancer use a variety of types of thermal energy as listed here:

- Radiofrequency (RF)[7]
- Laser[8]
- Focused ultrasound[9]
- Cryotherapy[10]
- Focused microwaves[11,12]

All of the preceding techniques have demonstrated some success in achieving ablation of breast cancer tumors—currently all of these techniques would be considered work-in-progress for breast cancer treatments. **Figure 1.1** depicts a thermotherapy scale in which the approximate range of temperature for each treatment modality is given. In the case of RF, laser, and ultrasound ablative procedures, high temperatures typically greater than 60°C are used in destroying the tumor tissue. With RF, laser, ultrasound, and cryotherapy for tumor ablation, the invasive cancer tumor size treated is typically less than 1.5 to 2 cm in maximum dimension as described by Huston and Simmons.[4] In contrast, because of selective microwave heating properties of breast carcinomas, transcutaneous FMT could be used to treat small to large invasive cancer tumors up to about 8 cm in maximum tumor dimension, as this book will show.

This book concentrates on the clinical rationale, physics, preclinical and clinical results for the minimally invasive treatment of breast cancer by elevation of the breast cancer tumor temperature to the range of about 43° to 52°C using wide-field focused microwaves. Clinical data presented demonstrate that temperatures in the range of about 48° to 50°C might provide the desired therapeutic range in preoperative transcutaneous focused microwave heat-alone treatment of invasive breast cancers in the intact breast. Clinical data also demonstrate that lower-temperature 43° to 46°C focused microwave thermotherapy might be used preoperatively in a combination treatment with preoperative chemotherapy for treating large primary invasive breast cancer tumors.

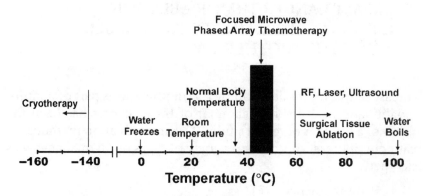

Figure 1.1 Thermotherapy scale showing the approximate range of temperatures for tumor ablation methods.

The general situation for heating a tumor (cancerous or benign) within tissue by means of a noninvasive heat-delivering source is depicted in **Figure 1.2**. The fundamental problem of transcutaneous heat delivery is to elevate the tumor temperature without burning the intervening tissue, primarily the superficial tissue layers. With transcutaneous heat delivery, the higher the required tumor temperature, the higher the risk of burning the intervening superficial tissues. Furthermore, breast carcinomas and tumor cells in the margins often follow the shape of irregular three-dimensional contours, with tumor distribution in the ducts or invasion into surrounding tissues; a well-defined circular or elliptical ablation zone is not always appropriate or sufficient for treating the entire tumor bed. As is described in detail in this book, a focused microwave phased array (FMPA) of multiple radiating sources directs its radiated energy at the tumor as depicted conceptually in **Figure 1.3**. An adaptive phased array thermotherapy system[13] using multiple transcutaneous radiating sources to produce RF energy or focused microwave energy is depicted in **Figure 1.4**. In this general case, a minimally invasive electric-field probe sensor needle monitors the microwave field in the tumor and provides a feedback signal to a microwave receiver and signal processing computer that adaptively controls the phase (timing) of the coherent array radiating sources to rapidly and reliably focus the microwave energy and induced heat in the tumor region. The amplitude/power level of the radiating sources is adjusted to achieve a desired tumor temperature.

Transcutaneous FMPA thermotherapy technology is a promising approach for use in breast conservation because it can preferentially heat and damage high-water-, high-ion-content breast carcinomas over an arbitrary narrow to wide region of the breast, compared to lesser degrees of heating that can occur in lower-water-, lower-ion-content adipose and glandular breast tissues.[14] At present, RF, laser, and ultrasound ablation methods might be limited in their effectiveness, particularly for breast tumors larger than about 2 cm measured by ultrasound, because each of these methods tends to ablate a well-defined limited elliptical or spherical volume of tissue and does not fully treat the tumor cells in margins that can extend to a diameter of 6 to 8 cm or more. In practice, tumor or tissue treatment volume (denoted V) can be computed approximately according to the equation of an ellipsoid:

$$V = 0.542\,LWD \tag{1.1}$$

where the three orthogonal tumor diameters, or tissue diameters, are L = length, W = width, and D = depth. By Equation 1.1, a well-defined 2-cm-diameter spherical tumor has a volume of 4.2 cc, and a 2-cm uniform surgical margin around the tumor (that is, 6-cm [spherical] total tissue diameter including the tumor and margin) produces an ex-

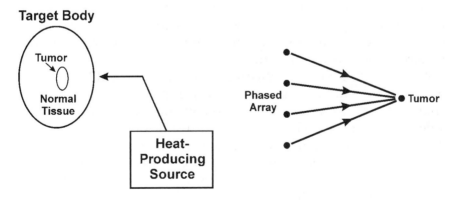

Figure 1.2   General problem of heating a deep-seated tumor by using an external heating source.

Figure 1.3   A phased array of energy sources focuses on a tumor target.

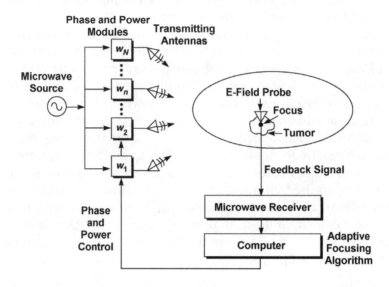

Figure 1.4   General case of multiple transcutaneous radiating sources delivering adaptively focused radiofrequency or microwave energy to a deep tumor in tissue.

cised tissue volume of 113.2 cc, or 27 times the tumor volume itself. For the same 2-cm-size spherical tumor, a 3-cm surgical margin (8-cm spherical tissue diameter) would produce an excised tissue volume of 268.3 cc, or 64 times the tumor volume itself. Therefore, in these two simple examples, a large treatment volume is potentially required in ablating the visible tumor and the microscopic cancer cells in the tumor margins. Heating large tissue volumes containing breast carcinomas or benign tumors is the hypothesis under investigation for focused microwave breast thermotherapy.

An artist's concept of a transcutaneous wide-field FMPA thermotherapy treatment of the breast is depicted in **Figure 1.5**. The term *array* here refers to two or more microwave applicators positioned in a desired fashion to deliver the desired treatment field, which produces the desired elevated temperature in the tumor. The term *phased* refers to an adjustment in the timing of the electromagnetic waves generated by the microwave applicators to produce a focused (concentrated) microwave field.

As described in detail in Chapter 3, in a focused microwave thermotherapy treatment the breast is compressed and dual air-cooled microwave applicators with large apertures surround the breast in a mammography fashion. The idea for treating the breast in this particular manner came about while I was already performing research in the field of FMTC,[13] and I then began reviewing the subjects of mammography and breast needle biopsy methodology. Breast compression, in particular, reduces the penetration depth for the microwaves and reduces the blood flow in the tumor region, allowing rapid heating of the tumor. An interstitial microwave needle probe, placed under ultrasound guidance, is used to measure the focal microwave power, which provides a required feedback signal to focus the microwaves at the tumor site. In general, it is not possible to focus microwave energy reliably on a breast tumor in heterogeneous breast tissues unless a feedback probe in the tumor is used in combination with a focusing algorithm.

An interstitial temperature sensor monitors the tumor temperature during FMT treatment to provide feedback for microwave power control. For breast thermotherapy, the two breast compression plates are made of a microwave-transparent plastic material that is sufficiently rigid to compress the breast but is not heated significantly by the microwaves. A suitably sized rectangular aperture is provided in each of

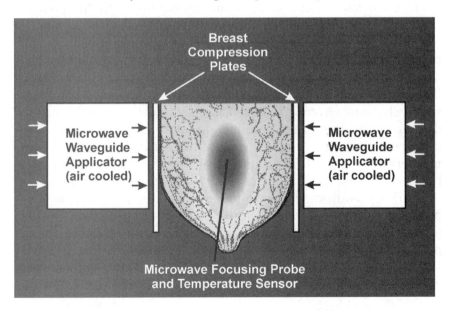

Figure 1.5   Artist's depiction of externally applied wide-field focused microwave phased array thermotherapy treatment of cancer in the intact breast.

Source: Molecular Medicine Today, O'Brien, C., Hyperthermia: getting tumours to feel the heat, P48, 1996, with permission from Elsevier.

the compression plates to allow airflow to reach the skin and to allow a standard ultrasound transducer to locate the tumor and accurately place the microwave probe and temperature probe in the tumor. The artist's concept of the microwave treatment field in Figure 1.5 is depicted as a wide region in the breast and is intended to provide heating to both the primary breast cancer tumor and any microscopic tumor cells in the margins—this wide-field focused microwave selective heating approach is considered a significant advantage over other ablation methods that can achieve only localized heating over a limited region.

As demonstrated in Chapter 4 by computer simulations and in Chapter 5 by phantom measurements, the actual shape of the microwave heating field is dependent on the water content and ion content of the tissues exposed to the focused microwaves. Malignant breast tumors and other breast lesions tend to have high water and high ion content, allowing the possibility for preferential tumor heating in the presence of lower-water- and lower-ion-content normal breast tissues such as fat, glandular, ductal, and connective tissues in the breast.

Phantom tests of the focused microwave breast thermotherapy technique confirming selective breast tumor heating (for simulated breast tumors of variable number and size in simulated normal breast tissue) and animal tests confirming safety are discussed in Chapter 5. Human clinical Phase I safety (Gardner et al[11]) and Phase II efficacy (Vargas et al[12]) studies, described in Chapters 6 and 7, respectively, have been conducted to demonstrate safety and to determine the minimum required thermal dose for focused microwaves to heat and completely kill primary invasive breast carcinomas prior to surgery. The temperatures administered to invasive breast cancers with transcutaneous focused microwaves in the safety and efficacy studies were in the range of 43° to 52°C, with an emphasis for preoperative heat-alone treatment in the range of 48° to 50°C for maximum treatment effectiveness and safety. This temperature range is in contrast with other thermal ablation methods (RF, laser, and focused ultrasound), which generally use temperatures between 60° and 100°C to ablate breast cancers (refer to Figure 1.1). As discussed in Chapter 2, in vitro data from the literature demonstrate that tumor cell kill depends on the induced tumor temperature and the duration of heating.

A number of possible indications of use for FMT can be hypothesized for invasive breast cancers where breast conservation is indicated. For example, preoperative thermotherapy could be considered in the following three possible protocols:

Protocol 1: Use preoperative FMT to reduce the rate of positive margins and reduce the rate of second surgery (reincision) when used with standard breast conservation (wide-excision lumpectomy followed by radiation therapy).

Protocol 2: Use preoperative FMT to eliminate the need for breast surgery if all of the breast cancer cells can be completely destroyed; follow-up with radiation therapy.

Protocol 3: Use preoperative FMT followed by surgery alone. A number of clinical studies have been exploring the use of 4 to 5 fractions of postoperative localized radiation therapy restricted to the tumor mass and margins instead of conventional full-breast irradiation administered in 20 to 30 fractions.[15] FMT in 1 to 3 fractions prior to surgery might be able to play a similar role in sterilizing the localized tumor mass and margins without the numerous side effects of radiation therapy given post surgery.

It is unlikely that protocol 2 or 3 would be attempted until protocol 1 is investigated and proved in randomized clinical trials. In protocol 1, as depicted in **Figure 1.6**, thermotherapy would be used prior to BCS and radiation therapy and should not place the patient at higher risk for breast cancer recurrence or significant added side effects compared to standard breast conservation. Primary end points for protocol 1 could be margin status (positive, close, or negative) at the time of initial surgery, rate of second incisions, and long-term (5 to 10 years) follow-up for rate of local recurrences of breast cancer. Chapter 8 describes the results of a randomized study of preoperative FMT that begins to investigate protocol 1. Other potential clinical research studies for focused microwave treatment of various stages of breast cancer, breast cancer prevention, and treatment of benign breast lesions are outlined in Chapter 10. The next section focuses on understanding the importance of tumor margins in breast cancer.

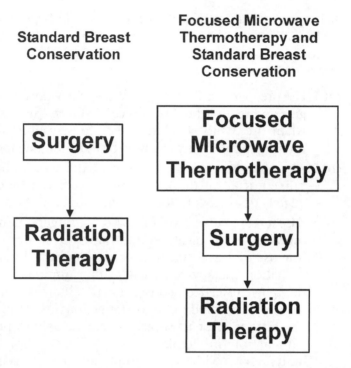

Figure 1.6 Standard breast conservation protocol compared to a new protocol in which preoperative focused microwave phased array thermotherapy is administered prior to breast conservation.

1.3 THE IMPACT OF TUMOR MARGINS IN BREAST CANCER

Published studies show that the rate of close or positive margins and rate of reexcision during breast conservation surgery can be substantial. For example, a 10-year study performed at Dartmouth and Beth Israel Deaconess Medical Center between 1990 and 1999 involved 546 lumpectomies as described by Gibson et al.[16] Invasive breast cancer was found in 83% of the lumpectomy specimens, and the remaining 17% of specimens had ductal carcinoma in situ. Of these 546 lumpectomies, 301 (55%) patients had positive or close margins, and these patients underwent reexcision. It was noted that the rate of reexcision during this 10-year study remained fairly constant at about 50%.

Another study was performed at M. D. Anderson Cancer Center in Houston, Texas, between 1970 and 1994 and involved 1153 consecutive breast cancer patients with stage I and stage II breast cancer as described by Mirza et al.[17] For this 24-year study, patients with positive or unknown margins at pathologic examination from the lumpectomy specimens resulted in a 39% reexcision rate. In another study, by the European Organization for Research and Treatment of Cancer (EORTC), with patient enrollment between 1989 and 1996, surgical excision of the primary tumor with a 1-cm margin of macroscopically normal tissue (lumpectomy) was performed for 5318 patients with a reported reexcision rate of 24.6%.[18] Patients were eligible for the EORTC study with clinical tumors T1 (tumor 0- to 2-cm diameter) or T2 (tumor >2-cm and ≥5-cm diameter), N0 or N1 (clinically node negative or positive), and M0 (no metastasis). In the EORTC study, any removal of additional breast tissue after the excision of the primary tumor was termed a reexcision, whether it was performed during the same surgical session or later. Therefore, from the preceding three studies, the rate of reexcision for breast carcinomas was in the range of 25% to 55%.

As depicted in **Figure 1.7**, in current surgical practice for breast cancer, in wide-excision lumpectomy (also referred to as partial mastectomy or quadrantectomy) an approximate 2- to 3-cm margin of "normal" tissue surrounding the elliptically shaped tumor mass is removed to achieve negative margins as described by Newman.[19] Thus, depending on breast tumor size, the maximum dimension of a wide excision can vary from as small as about 4 cm for small tumors to as large as about 10 cm or more for large tumors. *Therefore, any new treatment procedure for breast cancers should be capable of treating small and/or large arbitrary-shaped regions of the breast, up to about 10 cm in maximum dimension, that contain the breast tumor mass and the tumor cells in the margins. Ideally, the treatment volume of any new treatment modality should be matched with the volume containing the tumor mass and margins. Furthermore, the treatment zone volume of any new breast cancer treatment must not compromise the ability to perform sentinel lymph node mapping and biopsy and should have limited side effects.*

Intraoperative pathology consultation is typically used to ensure that the margins are negative for carcinomas prior to completing the first surgical procedure. During wide-excision lumpectomy, the surgical specimen is commonly marked with multicolor ink to identify the medial, lateral, superior, inferior, anterior, and posterior aspects

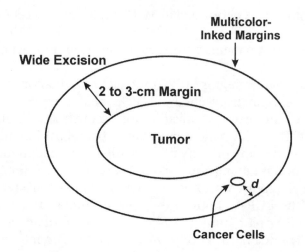

Figure 1.7   Depiction of wide-excision lumpectomy in which a 2 to 3-cm margin of tissue surrounding the tumor is removed.

of the breast tissue.[19,20] The multicolor ink technique reduces the amount of tissue that has to be reexcised to achieve negative margins should tumor cells be found at or near specific margins during the first excision. Typically, during lumpectomy with intraoperative pathology consultation, the initial surgical specimen is examined (often using the frozen section technique) for tumor cells at or near the margins while the patient remains in the operating room. If tumor cells (either invasive or intraductal) are found close to (for example, less than 1 mm from) the inked margins, the pathologist will recommend to the surgeon that additional tissue be excised at the involved inked margin (sometimes referred to as *surgical shaving*) as shown in **Figure 1.8**.

A final diagnosis by permanent section pathology can more accurately identify tumor cells at or near the margins, which can necessitate a second surgical procedure (second incision). Both the amount of breast tissue excised relative to the size of the breast and the use of a second incision have an impact on the breast cosmetic result,[19-24] and it is desirable for cosmetic reasons to avoid a second incision. Cosmesis also depends on the size and location of the tumor. For example, tumors located medially tend to have poorer cosmetic results

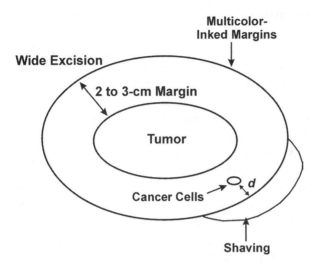

Figure 1.8   Depiction of a surgical shaving at an inked edge in which tumor cells are pathologically found close to or at the multicolor-inked surgical edge.

compared to laterally located tumors.[21] Clinical results indicate that significantly less breast tissue is excised for T1 tumors compared to T2 tumors.[23] The amount of skin removed in the first lumpectomy is usually quantified by the size of an ellipse given by length L and width W. If a second incision is required, the incision usually encompasses the original skin incision length (L in millimeters) plus about 2 mm in width. Thus, for a second incision the typical amount of skin excised is on the order of $L \times 4$ mm^2.

Singletary[20] has recently reviewed in detail the impact of breast tumor margins on locoregional recurrence. Margins are commonly described in terms of positive, close, and negative as follows: a *positive* margin refers to breast tumor cells located at the surgical margin. *Close* margin often refers to breast tumor cells located at a distance 1 mm or less from the surgical margin. *Negative* margin often refers to breast tumor cells located at a distance greater than 1 mm from the surgical margin. In some clinical studies, negative margin widths as large as 5 mm have been used as a criterion for judging whether a margin is close or negative. For the case of positive, 1-mm, and 2-mm negative margin widths, there is a significantly higher locoregional recurrence rate, with 5 to 10 years follow-up, when tumor cells are found at the surgical margin (positive margin) compared to when there is a negative margin. For example, when the negative margin width was taken as > 1 mm, five studies (Singletary, Table 1)[20] of 1375 patients with invasive breast cancer, receiving breast conservation therapy with 57 to 127 months follow-up showed that the mean locoregional recurrence rate for positive margins was 16.2% versus 2.6% for negative margins as depicted in **Figure 1.9**.[20] A subset of these clinical studies investigated negative, close, and positive margins. For example when the negative margin width was defined as > 1 mm, the mean local recurrence rates of three studies (Singletary, Table 2)[20] with 45 to 123 months follow-up were 4.3%, 6.6%, and 19% for negative, close, and positive margins, respectively. In these clinical studies the amount of radiation varies from 45 to 72.5 Gy (including radiation boost in some cases), some patients receive chemotherapy, and some patients receive tamoxifen. In addition to surgical margin status, significant independent predictors of locoregional recurrence include age (< 50 years), large tumor size, positive lymph nodes, not receiving chemotherapy, and not receiving hormonal therapy (Tamoxifen).[17] A problem encountered

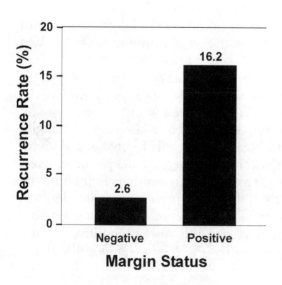

Figure 1.9 A comparison of the local recurrence rates, with 5- to 10-year follow-up, for patients with invasive breast cancer receiving breast conservation treatment and having positive or negative margins (1-mm margin width)

Source: Raw data in Singletary, Table 1.[20]

with positive margins is the hypoxic environment of the surgical scar bed, which provides an inherent tumor cell resistance to radiation therapy,[19] again suggesting the need for additional or alternative treatment modalities such as FMT.

1.4 BREAST CANCER: RATES FOR BREAST CONSERVATION THERAPY AND MASTECTOMY

In 1991, there was a consensus of opinion that breast conservation treatment (lumpectomy plus radiation therapy) could be used to treat up to 80% of new breast cancers.[25] In 1992, the American College of Surgeons' survey of 41,000 tumor registry patients indicated that only 25.5% were treated by breast conservation.[26] A review of more than 36,000 Medicare patients revealed that, on average, 12.1% were treated with breast conservation and 87.9% were treated with mastectomy.[27] Furthermore, the study reported geographic variations in the use of BCS and radiation in Medicare patients, with the frequency ranging from 3.5% to 21.2% in various states. Starting in 1990 (the year of the National Institutes of Health Consensus Conference—Early Stage Breast Cancer), the use of BCS increased annually; by 1995, 60% of women with stage I and 39% of women with stage II breast cancer received breast conservation treatment. Regional variation in breast conservation was observed (stage I breast cancer, range 41.4–71.4%; stage II breast cancer, range 23.8–48.0%), indicating barriers to widespread adoption of the Consensus Conference recommendations.[28]

Estimates of new cases of breast cancer in the year 2005 in the United States included 211,240 cases of invasive breast cancer and 58,490 new cases of in situ breast cancer, or a total of 269,730 new cases of breast cancer.[29] Based on 2004 US Census Bureau statistics,[30] the overall female population is expected to increase from 144 million in 2000 (150 million in 2005 by interpolation) to 171 million by 2020, and to 185 million in 2030, representing an increase in female population of 28.5% in 30 years. The percent of elderly female population (defined as 65 years and older) was 14.2% (20.5 million) in 2000, 14.7% (22 million) in 2005, and is expected to increase to 18.1% (31 million) in 2020 and to 21.6% (40 million) in 2030, representing a doubling of the elderly female population in 30 years due to the aging of the baby boomer generation. The elderly female population has a high incidence rate of breast cancer.[29] Thus, new cases of breast cancer, invasive and in situ, likely will rise annually for many years to come and breast conservation techniques will continue to be an important component of patient care. In current clinical practice, the percentage of patients treated with breast conservation is lower than expected; therefore, breast conservation therapy is underutilized in the United States, with rates ranging from 10% to 45% depending on patient age, treatment in the northeast versus southern regions, affluent socioeconomic status, treatment in metropolitan areas at a cancer center or teaching hospital, and lower reimbursement rates for lumpectomy codes.[19]

Given the present 45% or lower rate of BCS procedures practiced in the United States, improved treatments that could encourage a higher utilization of breast conservation are desirable. In some cases, patients do not want to undergo radiation therapy[31] and an alternate treatment, such as FMT, to sterilize the tumor bed, can be a viable approach without significant added side effects.

1.5 USE OF PREOPERATIVE THERMOCHEMO-THERAPY FOR DOWNSIZING LARGE BREAST CARCINOMAS

The prognosis for patients with large primary breast carcinomas in the intact breast is highly dependent on their clinical and histopathologic stage at diagnostic presentation. In addition to low survival rates, patients with large breast cancer tumors can require extensive surgical procedures that range from mastectomy alone to mastectomy followed by reconstructive surgery. Various regimens of chemotherapy are administered to breast cancer patients to treat systemic cancer to attempt to provide improved disease-free survival as well as overall survival.[32,33]

As discussed in this section, chemotherapy agents (particularly the anthracyclines doxorubicin and epirubicin) are often used in the treatment of large breast carcinomas. The expression *locally advanced breast cancer* (LABC) is sometimes used to categorize large breast carcinomas.[34] However, there is no standard definition for LABC, and in this section I simply use the phrases "large breast carcinomas" and "large breast cancer tumors." The aim of neoadjuvant (primary) systemic treatment for large breast cancer tumors is to improve surgical options—in particular, to downsize tumors so that BCS can be used instead of mastectomy.[33] Thermotherapy is known to enhance the cytotoxic effects of chemotherapy. This section describes the combination of thermotherapy with anthracycline-based chemotherapy and standard of care for improved treatment of breast cancer.

Over the last 25 years, the anthracycline chemotherapy agent doxorubicin has been commonly used to treat breast cancer in many of the large clinical studies performed by the NSABP. **Table 1.1** lists all of the NSABP protocols in which doxorubicin has been used in combination with other chemotherapy agents, with the accrual dates and the total subject accrual. Doxorubicin and epirubicin are anthracycline chemotherapy agents that are commonly considered a base part of standard of care when chemotherapy is recommended for treatment of breast cancer.[33]

Note that in the ongoing NSABP B-36 protocol, the anthracycline epirubicin (also known as epidoxorubicin) was included in the new arm of 6 cycles of FEC (fluorouracil, epirubicin, cyclophosphamide) compared to the control arm of 4 cycles of AC (doxorubicin and cyclophosphamide) in a postoperative setting for patients with histologically negative axillary nodes.

Recent treatment approaches have used chemotherapy regimens in a preoperative setting to reduce tumor size and increase the rate of breast conservation (partial mastectomy or lumpectomy) for patients with large breast cancer tumors. For example, in the NSABP B-18 randomized trial, the impact on survival for primary preoperative AC chemotherapy was studied in women with operable breast cancer.[35–37] Although there was no improvement in survival when AC chemotherapy was given preoperatively compared to postoperatively (survival at 9 years was 69% preoperative versus 70% postoperative),[37] there was an improvement in the use of breast conservation. In NSABP B-18, a total of 1523 patients were enrolled with 65% of patients already breast conservation candidates and 35% candidates only for mastectomy at the time of enrollment. A complete clinical tumor (breast and axilla) response was achieved in 17% of patients, and a partial

Table 1.1   List of NSABP Protocols That Have Included the Anthracycline doxorubicin Chemotherapy Agent as Part of the Study.

NSABP Breast Protocol with Doxorubicin (Adriamycin)	Dates Open and Closed to Accrual	Total Subject Accrual
B-11	1981–1984	707
B-12	1981–1984	1106
B-15	1984–1988	2338
B-16	1984–1989	1296
B-18	1988–1993	1523
B-22	1989–1991	2305
B-23	1991–1998	2008
B-25	1992–1994	2548
B-27	1995–2000	2411
B-28	1995–1998	3060
B-29	1997–1999	893
B-30	1999–2004	5351
B-31	2000–2005	2130
B-36	2004–present	(goal = 2700)
B-38	2004–present	(goal = 4800)
Total = 15 studies	**Time Period = 1981 to Present**	**Total = 35,176 (including goal)**

Source: NSABP Protocol Chart, April 2006, http://www.nsabp.pitt.org.

response in 58% of patients was achieved for an overall response rate of 75%. In the B-18 study, 69 of 256 (27%) patients for whom a mastectomy had been planned before randomization to preoperative chemotherapy were converted to breast conservation, and 10 of 69 (14.5%) of these patients had an ipsilateral (same breast) breast tumor recurrence.[36] Tumor size reduction and size of the breast are highly significant for predicting when breast conservation can be performed. Complete pathologic tumor response, in the breast and axilla, is a prognostic marker for both disease-free survival and overall survival. In NSABP B-18, for tumors with a complete clinical response, 26% of the tumors also had a complete pathologic response.

In the NSABP B-18 study before randomization, clinical (palpable) tumor size and clinical nodal status influenced the surgeon's decision to recommend lumpectomy or mastectomy. Patient age was not a factor in the decision to propose lumpectomy. In the B-18 study, there was an indication that many physicians considered lumpectomy inappropriate for node-positive patients before randomization; however, it is now known that clinical node status is a poor measure of pathologic nodal status. For the B-18 study, 48% of patients with clinically negative nodes were actually pathologically node positive, and 14% of patients with clinically positive nodes were pathologically node negative.

In NSABP B-18, before randomization, mastectomy was proposed in 35% of patients overall in the preoperative chemotherapy group. The proposal to recommend mastectomy before randomization depended on tumor size and clinical nodal status. In the B-18 study, there were 29% T1 tumors (0 to 2 cm), 58% T2 tumors (>2 to ≥5 cm), and 13% T3 tumors (>5 cm) based on clinical examination (palpation). In the B-18 study, 74% of patients were node negative and 26% of patients were node positive. For T2 tumors, mastectomy was recommended in 32% of patients overall (68% proposed rate of lumpectomy prior to treatment), and for T3 tumors, mastectomy was recommended in 97% of patients overall (3% proposed rate of lumpectomy prior to treatment).

After preoperative chemotherapy was administered, for T2 tumors, mastectomy was performed in 29% of patients (71% rate of lumpectomy), and for T3 tumors, mastectomy was performed in 78% of patients (22% rate of lumpectomy). If the axillary nodes were clinically negative, mastectomy was proposed in 29% of patients overall, and if the axillary nodes were clinically positive, mastectomy was proposed in 51% of patients overall. After preoperative chemotherapy was administered, the rate of mastectomy was not affected for originally node-negative patients, but was reduced from 51% to 41% for originally node-positive patients. The greatest change in the rate of mastectomy occurred for patients with T3 tumors (either node negative or node positive before randomization). Preoperative chemotherapy reduced the rate of mastectomy for T3, node-negative patients from 96% (proposed) to 86% (actual) and for T3, node-positive patients from 98% (proposed) to 67% (actual).

The combination of Adriamycin (doxorubicin) and Cytoxan (cyclophosphamide) is one of the chemotherapy regimens administered to patients with advanced breast cancer for systemic treatment and for downsizing large breast cancer tumors. From the NSABP B-18 study results discussed earlier, preoperative AC is known to reduce the size of operable breast tumors, and in some cases mastectomy patients can be converted to breast conservation patients. AC chemotherapy is commonly administered intravenously in four cycles with each cycle lasting 21 days. Patients undergoing preoperative AC receive all four cycles of AC, unless locoregional progressive disease occurs before completion of therapy. The remaining courses can be administered postoperatively to patients who develop clinically progressive disease during chemotherapy. Women whose tumors become inoperable during therapy are listed as treatment failures and are managed at the discretion of their physicians. In NSABP B-18, all patients 50 years of age or older received tamoxifen 10 mg twice a day for 5 years, beginning on the day after their last dose of chemotherapy.

Another large study of preoperative chemotherapy is NSABP B-27 in which women with operable breast cancer were randomly assigned to three groups to receive four cycles of preoperative AC followed by surgery, four cycles of preoperative AC followed by four cycles of preoperative docetaxel (an antitubulin), or four cycles of preoperative AC followed by surgery and four cycles of docetaxel as described by Bear et al.[38] The large NSABP B-27 study enrolled 2411 patients, and results of the study indicate that the complete pathologic response rate increased from 12.9% in the preoperative AC-alone arm to 26.1% in the preoperative AC preoperative docetaxel arm. However, the rate of breast conservation and overall survival was not affected by the administration of docetaxel.

Though the results of large clinical trials such as the NSABP B-18 and B-27 studies are encouraging in terms of tumor response, these results indicate that a significant improvement in neoadjuvant treatment methodology is desirable.

As discussed in Section 1.2, breast cancer tumor ablation with RF,[7] interstitial laser photocoagulation,[8] focused ultrasound,[9] cryotherapy,[10] or focused microwaves[11,12] as part of a multimodality approach in the treatment of breast cancer is a subject of recent interest.[4-6] A Phase I safety study of focused microwaves[11] for 10 mastectomy-eligible patients, with mean clinical tumor size of 4.19 cm (range 0.9 to 8.0 cm) at enrollment, demonstrated tumor shrinkage and/or tumor cell kill in 8 of 10 (80%) patients as a result of a single thermotherapy treatment.

A Phase II dose-escalation study (Vargas et al[12]) of heat-alone thermotherapy, prior to surgery, using externally applied focused microwave phased array treatment of primary breast cancer in 25 patients with early-stage tumors demonstrated that a cumulative equivalent minutes tumor thermal dose of 210 minutes or greater (relative to 43°C) is predictive of 100% necrosis for invasive breast carcinomas. The Phase II dose-escalation study also demonstrated that preoperative focused microwave breast thermotherapy does not impair the ability to perform sentinel lymph node mapping as described by Vargas et al.[39] Microwave energy is promising because it can preferentially heat and damage high-water-, high-ion-content breast carcinomas, compared to lesser degrees of heating that occurs in lower-water-, lower-ion-content adipose and glandular tissues.[14,40]

The clinical rationale for the use of thermotherapy and chemotherapy has been established in prior studies.[41-43] The application of thermotherapy provides tumor cell kill by direct thermal cytotoxicity above 42.5°C and by thermal chemosensitization in the range of about 40°C to 44°C as demonstrated primarily in tissue cultures. These studies indicate a multiprocess synergism in cytotoxicity when thermotherapy (about 42°C to 44°C) is combined with the chemotherapy agent doxorubicin.[41-43] The drug doxorubicin gets into cells more easily at 43°C compared to 37°C, possibly because of a change in the plasma membrane at the higher temperature, and doxorubicin cytotoxicity can be enhanced at 43°C when the tumors are heated longer than 60 minutes.[44]

Cyclophosphamide has also been demonstrated to be potentiated by thermotherapy. For example, increased cell kill was measured for cyclophosphamide (using EMT-6 mammary carcinoma in Balb/C mice) administered at temperatures of 40.5°C and, as the temperature was increased to 42°C, additional cell kill was observed.[41] Maximum effectiveness of heat and drug can be achieved when the heat is given about 4 hours after chemotherapy.[41] For patients with large breast tumors, the combination of FMT and neoadjuvant chemotherapy could improve tumor response rates, increase the use of breast conservation, and reduce ipsilateral breast tumor recurrence.

Other drug combinations besides AC (NSABP B-18)[35-37] and AC with docetaxel (NSABP B-27)[38] have been considered for neoadjuvant treatment of breast cancer. Most combinations use the common base drug doxorubicin (anthracycline). **Table 1.2** summarizes the most common drug combinations that have used anthracyclines (doxorubicin or epirubicin) for preoperative treatment of breast cancer.[32,33]

Table 1.2   Drug Combinations that Use an Anthracycline for Neoadjuvant Treatment of Breast Cancer

Doxorubicin, cyclophosphamide (AC)
Doxorubicin, cyclophosphamide, cocetaxel (AC docetaxel)
Doxorubicin, cyclophosphamide, 5-fluorouracil (FAC)
Doxorubicin, cyclophosphamide, 5-fluorouracil (FAC), paclitaxel
Doxorubicin, paclitaxel (AP)
Doxorubicin, cyclophosphamide, vincristine, paclitaxel (CVAP)
Doxorubicin, cyclophosphamide, paclitaxel (ACP)
5-Fluorouracil, epirubicin, cyclophosphamide (FEC)
Paclitaxel, 5-fluorouracil, epirubicin, cyclophosphamide (FEC), Herceptin (tastuzumab)

Some of these drug combinations include 5-fluorouracil with AC (FAC), paclitaxel with FAC, paclitaxel with FEC and Herceptin (common name trastuzumab), doxorubicin and paclitaxel (Taxol), AC and paclitaxel, and cyclophosphamide, vincristine, Adriamycin (doxorubicin), and paclitaxel. The number of cycles of drug can vary from 3 to 12 cycles; the interval between cycles can vary from 14 days to 28 days; the drugs can be delivered in combination or sequentially.

A recent small study for HER-2 (human epidermal growth factor receptor 2) positive patients with T1, T2, T3, and T4 tumors explored the neoadjuvant drug combination of paclitaxel followed by FEC and Herceptin. A high rate of complete pathologic response (65.2%, $n = 23$) was reported by Buzdar et al,[45] but without an increase in breast conservation. For those patients that are HER-2 positive, Herceptin in combination with neoadjuvant chemotherapy as described earlier could be considered additionally in combination with preoperative thermochemotherapy.

In the past, breast cancer patients with distant metastases received breast surgery only to prevent local complications. A large majority of patients with metastases do not survive beyond 5 years after diagnosis—it is generally accepted in those cases that breast cancer surgery is palliative, and the primary treatment is systemic therapy with chemotherapy, hormonal treatment, and biologic therapy. However, a recently published nonrandomized study by Rapiti et al[46] has shown evidence that surgical removal of the primary tumor and achieving negative margins significantly improve patient survival: for 300 patients followed for 5 years, there was a 40% reduced risk of death for patients receiving surgery with negative margins compared to patients that did not receive surgery ($P = .049$). Therefore, for patients with distant metastases, the use of preoperative thermochemotherapy could contribute to an increase in negative margins and prevent additional metastasis of cancer cells, which could reduce the risk of death. Patients with and without distant metastases could benefit from preoperative thermochemotherapy.

1.6 SUMMARY

The incidence rate of smaller breast cancers tends to be increasing as increased screening and improved breast imaging technology is being developed. The number of new cases of breast cancer will increase steadily over the next 25 years due to increasing population and an older population in the United States. Peak prevalence might occur sometime in this period.[47] For breast cancer patients undergoing BCS procedures, it is critical to achieve negative margins to avoid an increased risk of local recurrence. Current wide-excision lumpectomy by itself sometimes does not eliminate all breast cancer cells from the margins. A presurgical focused microwave phased array thermotherapy treatment has been hypothesized to ablate cancer cells both in the primary tumor and in the tumor margins, which fundamentally requires a large effective heating field. Potential future indications of use for FMT to ablate early-stage invasive breast cancer cells prior to surgery to improve margins have been discussed. The use of breast conservation is currently underutilized. For large breast cancer tumors, preoperative FMT could be used in combination with standard-of-care preoperative chemotherapy to improve tumor response and potentially increase the use of breast conservation. The next chapter describes the interaction of microwave energy with breast tissues and breast lesions.

REFERENCES

1. Edney, JA. Breast cancer treatment for the future based on lessons from the past. *Am J Surg.* 2002;184:477–483.

2. Cady B, Stone MD, Schuler JG, et al. The new era in breast cancer: invasion, size, and nodal involvement dramatically decreasing as a result of mammographic screening. *Arch Surg.* 1996;131:301–308.

3. Fisher B, Anderson S, Bryant J, et al. Twenty-year follow-up of a randomized trial comparing total mastectomy, lumpectomy, and lumpectomy plus irradiation for the treatment of invasive breast cancer. *N Engl J Med.* 2002;347:1233–1241.

4. Huston TL, Simmons RM. Ablative therapies for the treatment of malignant diseases of the breast. *Am J Surg.* 2005;189:694–701.

5. Singletary ES. Minimally invasive techniques in breast cancer treatment. *Seminars in Surg Onc.* 2001;20:246–250.

6. Agnese DM, Burak WE. Ablative approaches to the minimally invasive treatment of breast cancer. *Cancer J.* 2005;11(1):77–82.

7. Fornage BD, Sneige N, Mirz AN, et al. Small (< 2-cm) breast cancer treated with US-guided radiofrequency ablation: feasibility study. *Radiology.* 2005;231: 215–224.

8. Dowlatshashi K, Francescatti DS, Bloom KJ. Laser therapy for small breast cancers. *Am J Surg.* 2002;184:359–363.

9. Huber PE, Jenne JW, Rastert R, et al. A new noninvasive approach in breast cancer therapy using magnetic resonance imaging-guided focused ultrasound surgery. *Cancer Res.* 2001;61:8441–8447.

10. Pfleiderer SO, Freesmeyer MG, Marx C, Kuhne-Heid R, Schneider A, Kaiser WA. Cryotherapy of breast cancer under ultrasound guidance: initial results and limitations. *Eur Radiol.* 2002;12:3009–3014.

11. Gardner RA, Vargas HI, Block JB, Vogel CL, Fenn AJ, Kuehl GV, Doval M. Focused microwave phased array thermotherapy for primary breast cancer. *Ann Surg Oncol.* 2002;9(4):326–332.

12. Vargas HI, Dooley WC, Gardner RA, Gonzalez KD, Vanegas R, Heywang-Kobrunner SH, Fenn AJ. Focused microwave phased array thermotherapy for ablation of early-stage breast cancer: results of thermal dose escalation. *Ann Surg Oncol.* 2004;11(2):139–146.

13. Fenn AJ, King GA. Adaptive radio-frequency hyperthermia-phased array system for improved cancer therapy: phantom target measurements. *Int J Hyperthermia.* 1994;10(2):189–208.

14. Joines WT, Zhang Y, Li C, Jirtle RL. The measured electrical properties of normal and malignant human tissues from 50 to 900 MHz. *Med Phys.* 1994;21(4): 547–550.

15. Arthur DW, Vicini FA. Accelerated partial breast irradiation as part of a breast conservation therapy. *J Clin Oncol.* 2005;23(8):1726–1735.

16. Gibson GR, Lesnikoski BA, Yoo J, Mott LA, Cady B, Barth RJ Jr. A comparison of ink-directed and traditional whole-cavity re-excision for breast lumpectomy specimens with positive margins. *Ann Surg Oncol.* 2001;8(9):693–704.

17. Mirza NQ, Vlastos G, Meric F, et al. Predictors of locoregional recurrence among patients with early-stage breast cancer treated with breast-conserving therapy. *Ann Surg Oncol.* 2002;9(3):256–265.

18. Bartelink H, Horiot J-C, Poortmans P, et al. Recurrence rates after treatment of breast cancer with standard radiation therapy and or without additional radiation. *N Engl J Med.* 2001;345:1378–1387.

19. Newman LA, Kuerer HM. Advances in breast conservation therapy. *J Clin Oncol.* 2005;23(8):1685–1697.

20. Singletary SE. Surgical margins in patients with early-stage breast cancer treated with breast conservation therapy. *Am J Surg.* 2002;184:383–393.

21. Cochrane RA, Valasiadou P, Wilson AR, Al-Ghazal SK, Macmillan RD. Cosmesis and satisfaction after breast-conserving surgery correlates with the percentage of breast volume excised. *Br J Surg.* 2003;90(12):1505–1509.

22. Rose MA, Olivotto IA, Cady B, et al. Conservative surgery and radiation therapy for early breast cancer. Long-term cosmetic results. *Arch Surg.* 1989;124: 153–157.

23. Wazer DE, DiPetrillo T, Schmidt-Ulrich R, Weld L, Marchant DJ, Robert NJ. Factors influencing cosmetic outcome and complication risk after conservative surgery and radiotherapy for early-stage breast carcinoma. *J Clin Oncol.* 1992;10:356–363.

24. Olivotto IA, Rose MA, Osteen RT, et al. Late cosmetic outcome after conservative surgery and radiotherapy: analysis of causes of cosmetic failure. *Int J Radiat Oncol Biol Phys.* 1989;17:747–753.

25. NIH Consensus Conference. Early stage breast cancer. *JAMA.* 1991;265:391–395.

26. Osteen TR, Steele GD Jr, Menck HR, Winchester DP. Regional difference in surgical management of breast cancer. *CA.* 1992;42(1):39–43.

27. Nattinger AB, Gottlieb MS, Veum J, Yahnke D, Goodwin JS. Geographic variation in the use of breast-conservation treatment for breast cancer. *N Engl J Med.* 1992;326(17):1102–1107.

28. Lazovich D, Solomon CC, Thomas DB, Moe RE, White E. Breast conservation therapy in the United States following the 1990 National Institutes of Health Consensus Development Conference on the treatment of patients with early stage invasive breast carcinoma. *Cancer.* 1999;86:628–637.

29. American Cancer Society. *Cancer Facts and Figures 2004.* Atlanta, Ga: American Cancer Society; 2004.

30. US Census Bureau. US Interim projections by age, sex, race, and hispanic origin. http://www.census.gov/ipc/www/usinterimproj. Accessed March 18, 2004.

31. Moelnaar S, Oort F, Sprangers M, et al. Predictors of patients' choices for breast-conserving therapy or mastectomy: a prospective study. *Br J Cancer.* 2004;90:2123–2130.

32. Hamilton A, Hortobagyi G. Chemotherapy: what progress in the last 5 years? *J Clin Oncol.* 2005;23(8):1760–1775.

33. Kaufmann M, Hortobagyi G, Goldhirsch A, et al. Recommendations from an international expert panel on the use of neoadjuvant (primary) systemic treatment of operable breast cancer. An update. *J Clin Oncol.* 2006:24(12):1940–1949.

34. Wolff AC, Davidson NE. Preoperative therapy in breast cancer: lessons from the treatment of locally advanced disease. *Oncologist.* 2002;7:239–245.

35. Fisher B, Brown A, Mamounas E. et al. Effect of preoperative chemotherapy on local-regional disease in women with operable breast cancer: findings from the National Surgical Adjuvant Breast and Bowel Project B-18. *J Clin Oncol.* 1997;15:2483–2493.

36. Fisher B, Bryant J, Wolmark N, et al. Effect of preoperative chemotherapy in the outcome of women with operable breast cancer. *J Clin Oncol.* 1998;16(8): 2672–2685.

37. Wolmark N, Wang J, Mamounas E, Bryant J, Fisher B. Preoperative chemotherapy in patients with operable breast cancer: nine-year results from National Surgical Adjuvant Breast and Bowel Project B-18. *J Natl Cancer Inst Monogr.* 2001;30:96–102.

38. Bear HD, Anderson S, Smith RE, et al. Sequential preoperative or postoperative docetaxel added to preoperative doxorubicin plus cyclophosphamide for operable breast cancer: National Surgical Adjuvant Breast and Bowel Project Protocol B-27. *J Clin Oncol.* 2006;24(13):2019–2027.

39. Vargas HI, Dooley WC, Gardner RA, Gonzalez KD, Heywang-Kobrunner SH, Fenn AJ. Success of sentinel lymph node mapping after breast cancer ablation with focused microwave phased array thermotherapy. *Am J Surg.* 2003;186: 330–332.

40. Campbell AM, Land DV. Dielectric properties of female human breast tissue measured in vitro at 3.2 GHz. *Phys Med Biol.* 1992;37(1):193–210.

41. Hornback N. *Hyperthermia and Cancer.* Boca Raton, Fla: CRC Press; 1984; I: 65–75, 94–104.

42. Dahl O, Mella O. Hyperthermia and chemotherapeutic agents. In: Field SB, Hand JW, eds. *An Introduction to the Practical Aspects of Clinical Hyperthermia.* New York: Taylor and Francis; 1990:chap 5,108–142.

43. Issels R. Clinical rationale for thermochemotherapy. In: Seegenschmiedt MH, Fessenden P, Vernon CC, eds. *Thermoradiotherapy and Thermochemotherapy.* Vol. 2. New York: Springer-Verlag; 1995; 2: chap 2, 25–33.

44. Urano M, Begley J, Reynolds R. Interaction between Adriamycin and hyperthermia: growth-phase-dependent thermal sensitization. *Int J Hyperthermia.* 1994;10(13):817–826.

45. Buzdar AU, Ibrahim NK, Francis D, et al. Significantly higher pathologic complete remission rate after neoadjuvant therapy with trastuzumab, paclitaxel, and epirubicin chemotherapy: Results of a randomized trial in human epidermal growth factor receptor 2-positive operable breast cancer. *J Clin Oncol* 2005;23(16):3676–3685.

46. Rapiti E, Verkooijen HM, Vlastos G, et al. Complete excision of primary breast tumor improves survival of patients with metastatic breast cancer at diagnosis. *J Clin Oncol.* 2006;24(18):2743–2749.

47. Verdecchia A, DeAngelis G, Capocaccia R. Estimation and projections of cancer prevalence from cancer registry date. *Statistics in Medicine.* 2002; 21:3511–3526.

Microwave Thermotherapy for Breast Cancer and Other Breast Lesions

2.1 INTRODUCTION

Mild thermotherapy (also known as *hyperthermia*), with induced tumor temperatures in the range of about 42°C to 46°C, is sometimes used in a multimodality cancer treatment regimen to enhance the effects of radiation therapy or chemotherapy. A large body of preclinical and clinical data has been published over the last three decades on this topic.[1-19] Cancer cells tend to be hypoxic (reduced oxygen content often caused by damaged tumor vasculature), which is a radioresistant characteristic that can limit the effectiveness of radiation therapy. Application of heat to cancerous tissue can improve the blood flow and oxygenation of the tissue and make radiation therapy more effective. In the case of chemotherapy, delivery of the chemotherapeutic agents to tumors through the bloodstream can be compromised by the damaged vasculature of the tumor region. When hyperthermia is applied to the cancerous tumor region, the blood vessels can expand; hence, the blood flow, and chemotherapy drug delivery, to the tumor can increase.

Common methods for delivering thermotherapy to tumors include interstitial[20] (percutaneous) applicators and external[21] (transcutaneous) applicators with either radiofrequency, ultrasound, or microwave energy. Heat-alone cancer treatment in the range of 42°C to 46°C, as used in some hyperthermia treatment protocols, would not be expected to provide 100% tumor cell kill; however, higher temperatures have been used in thermal ablation procedures to achieve complete tumor cell kill as described in Section 2.2. Theory for the interaction of microwave electric fields and tissue, in terms of heating, is then described briefly in Section 2.3. Microwave properties of breast tissues are described in Section 2.4.

2.2 HEAT-ALONE TREATMENT FOR BREAST CARCINOMAS

Thermal ablation has taken a prominent clinical research role in minimally invasive approaches that are being explored in the treatment of breast cancer.[22] Freezing of tumors can be achieved through cryoablation[23] (low temperature), whereas heat energy and tumor temperatures greater than 60°C (high temperature) can be generated by the use of interstitial laser photocoagulation,[24] radiofrequency-induced coagulation,[25] or focused ultrasound.[26] Moderate temperature ranges of about 48° to 52°C can be generated with transcutaneous focused microwave ablation[27] as described in this book.

The temperature range 48° to 52°C (moderate temperature) for transcutaneous focused microwave thermotherapy for breast cancer is of interest for two primary reasons: (1) in vitro cell survival experiments (reviewed later in this section) demonstrate significant or complete cell kill in the temperature range of about 48° to 52°C, and (2) the use of heat-alone transcutaneous focused microwave tumor treatment in the temperature range of 48° to 52°C appears to be safe (for avoiding burning of superficial tissues by the microwaves penetrating through the skin) and effective on treating breast carcinomas based on clinical studies as described in Chapters 6, 7, and 8.

The cytotoxic effects of hyperthermia alone using temperatures in the range of about 45°C to 53°C have been demonstrated on a variety of cell types in vitro.[28-30] In vitro studies by Gerhard et al demonstrated that human cell lines (HeLa and EB 33) can be significantly damaged by heat-alone treatment provided that temperatures in the range of at least 47° to 53°C can be achieved for sufficient time.[28] Note: The HeLa cells were a permanent cell line derived from human cervical carcinoma and the EB 33 cells were a permanent cell line derived from human prostatic carcinoma. As Gerhard shows, for EB 33 prostatic cells in vitro, no surviving cells were observed after 100 seconds (1.7 minutes) of exposure to 53°C heat alone.[9] Greater than 99% cell kill (within a 3-day period from the time of heat exposure) for EB 33 prostatic cells was obtained by heating at 47°C for 700 seconds (11.6 minutes) or at 49°C for 350 seconds (5.8 minutes). Example cell kill data based on the results from Gerhard are redrawn in **Figure 2.1** by using the following conversion: cell kill percentage = 100%-viable cell percentage. From Gerhard's data, little cell kill was achieved if the carcinoma was heated at 47°C for 4 minutes or less, whereas greater than 85% carcinoma cell kill occurred with 6 minutes of 47°C heating. When the temperature was increased to 49°C, little cell kill was observed with 1 minute of heating; however, 4 minutes of heating produced greater than 85% carcinoma cell kill. With a further increase of the tumor cell temperature to 53°C, little cell kill occurred if the heating time was only 30 seconds, but greater than 85% cell kill occurred when the heating time was at least 1.5 minutes. These heat-alone data are quantitative for determining a threshold temperature range and heating duration in which significant carcinoma cell kill occurs. Further study of Gerhard's data (Figure 2.1) shows that for 100% cell kill, about 6 minutes of heating at 49°C or about 12 minutes of heating at 47°C is required—it is estimated from these data that about 8 to 9 minutes of continuous heating at 48°C is required for 100% carcinoma cell kill.

Experimental studies by Sapareto and Dewey support the concept that tumor cell heating alone for 60 minutes at 43°C is tumoricidal, and the period of time to kill tumor cells decreases by a factor of 2 for each degree increase in temperature above about 43°C.[31] As described by Sapareto and Dewey,[31] thermal damage to tumors frequently exhibits a threshold-like response in which, once a certain

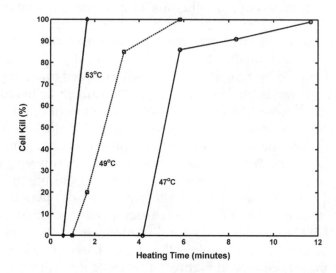

Figure 2.1 Percent cell kill, 2.5 days after thermotherapy treatment, for EB 33 prostatic cells in vitro, as a function of heating time at various temperatures (data were redrawn from Figure 1 of Gerhard[28]).

thermal dose is administered, only a slight increase in thermal dose can cause a large increase in tumor tissue damage. Some of the clinical studies of focused microwave thermotherapy reviewed in this book describe the empirical data used to identify a required minimum tumor thermal dose and minimum peak tumor temperature using focused microwave heating alone to induce 100% tumor cell kill (necrosis) for breast cancer. The next section briefly describes the interaction between microwaves and tissue.

2.3 MICROWAVE HEATING OF TISSUE

The interaction of a radiofrequency or microwave electromagnetic field (consisting of electric and magnetic field components) and tissue, and the resulting elevation of tissue temperature are fundamentally related to the complex permittivity (denoted here as ϵ_c) of the tissue.[32] The total electromagnetic field consists of an incident field and a scattered field, both of which are governed by Maxwell's equations. In vacuum (free space), microwaves (photons) travel at the speed of light, and in tissue, microwaves travel slower than the speed of light. In microwave hyperthermia, the electric-field component, denoted E with units of volts per meter, is a polarized vector quantity that applies a force (governed by the Lorentz force law) to dipole molecules, such as water, and to charges or ions present in the tissue. When the electric field is time varying (usually oscillating sinusoidally for hyperthermia treatments) in tissue, the applied force affects the water molecules and ions and they rotate, move, and collide with each other. The resulting microwave-induced molecular and ionic collisions produce heat energy, which in turn produces an elevation of the tissue temperature, particularly for high-water-, high-ion-content tissue. Mathematically, the complex relative permittivity consists of a real term that can be referred to as the relative "real" dielectric constant ϵ_{real} and an imaginary term that is termed the relative "imaginary" dielectric constant ϵ_{imag}. The complex permittivity of tissue can be expressed in terms of real and imaginary components as

$$\epsilon_c = \epsilon_0 (\epsilon_{real} - i\,\epsilon_{imag}) \qquad (2.1)$$

where ϵ_0 is the permittivity of vacuum (8.854×10^{-12} Farads per meter) and $i = \mathrm{sqrt}(-1)$ is the imaginary number. The real part of the dielectric constant of tissue affects primarily the wavelength of the electromagnetic radiation in the tissue (computation of the wavelength from measured dielectric parameters is discussed in Chapter 4, Section 4.3). The imaginary part of the dielectric constant affects primarily the electrical conductivity and the electromagnetic heating of tissue. The electrical (or ionic) conductivity (denoted σ with units of Siemens per meter) of tissue is expressed in terms of the imaginary part of the dielectric constant as

$$\sigma = 2\pi f \epsilon_0 \epsilon_{imag} \qquad (2.2)$$

where f is the frequency (units of cycles per second, or Hertz) of the microwave radiation. Data in the literature for tissue ionic conductivity are usually cited in units of either Siemens per meter (S/m) or milli-Siemens per centimeter (mS/cm)—the conversion between these two units is 1 mS/cm = 0.1 S/m, or 1 S/m = 10 mS/cm. In general, the dielectric parameters for tissue are temperature dependent:

the real part of the dielectric constant typically is reduced as temperature increases and the imaginary part of the dielectric constant typically increases as temperature increases. The microwave energy absorption per unit mass (or specific absorption rate [SAR] with units of watts per kilogram) of tissue is directly proportional to both the electrical conductivity σ of the tissue and the square of the magnitude of the applied electric field, denoted $|E|$, and is inversely proportional to the tissue density (denoted ρ with units of kg/m^3):

$$SAR = \frac{1}{2}\frac{\sigma}{\rho}|E|^2 \qquad (2.3)$$

The rise in temperature (ΔT) in a given time interval (Δt) with a given applied SAR is expressed as:

$$\Delta T = \frac{1}{c} SAR \, \Delta t \qquad (2.4)$$

where c is the specific heat capacity of the tissue, and thermal conduction and perfusion effects are ignored. The SAR and rise in temperature defined by Equations 2.3 and 2.4, respectively, are usually thought of in terms of macroscopic heating of a solid tumor mass of a given size. However, one can also consider these two equations on a microscopic level as being valid for the case of heating a single tumor cell. An individual high-water-, high-ion-content cancer cell embedded in low-water-content normal breast tissue should be rapidly heated and ablated when exposed to an intense microwave field.

As described in Section 2.2, microwave energy is a promising approach for breast thermotherapy because microwaves can preferentially heat and damage high-water-, high-ion-content breast carcinomas, compared to lesser degrees of heating that might occur in lower-water-, lower-ion-content adipose and breast glandular tissues. The fast oscillation of the microwave energy combined with the high water and high ion content and corresponding high electrical conductivity of breast carcinomas produces a significant amount of molecular and ionic friction in the breast carcinoma cells that generates heat and rapidly elevates the temperature of the tumor.

2.4 MICROWAVE CHARACTERISTICS OF NORMAL BREAST TISSUE, BREAST CANCER, AND BENIGN LESIONS

This section provides detailed measured data for microwave properties of breast tissue, including breast cancer and benign lesions. The presence of ions in breast cancer and in benign lesions is important because the ions contribute very significantly (in addition to water content) to how well tumors are heated by microwaves. Information on benign breast lesions is included because these lesions are common and it is essential to know how microwaves can affect any lesions in breast cancer patients—benign lesions might also be a candidate target lesion for microwave treatments.

A lateral view of the female breast[33] is shown in **Figure 2.2**. The amount of glandular and fatty tissue within the breast can vary widely among patients, from extremely dense glandular tissue in younger patients and primarily fatty tissue in older patients. Breast cancer cells usually form within the lactiferous ducts and glandular tissue lobules as described by Love.[34] Cells can be categorized as *well differentiated* (cells having normal functions), *moderately differentiated* (cells having less than normal function and that are cancerous), and *poorly differentiated* (cells having no useful function, that is, cancerous). The first indication of abnormal cell growth within the duct is referred to as *intraductal hyperplasia*, followed by *intraductal hyperplasia with atipia*. When the ducts become nearly full, the condition is known as *ductal carcinoma in situ* (DCIS). These three abnormal cell conditions are commonly referred to as precancers. Finally, when the ductal carcinomas break through the ductal wall, the lesion is referred to as *invasive ductal cancer*. Cancer forms in the same way in the glandular lobules of the breast. All of the cells mentioned previously are often cited as being high-water-content with the exception of pure fat tissue (low-water-content) and pure glandular/connective tissue (medium-water-content) within the breast.

The structure of the breast is described in detail by Haagensen.[35] The breast consists of epithelial parenchyma of acini and ducts and their supporting muscular and fascial elements, fat, blood vessels, nerves, lymphatics, and connective tissue. The epithelial parenchyma

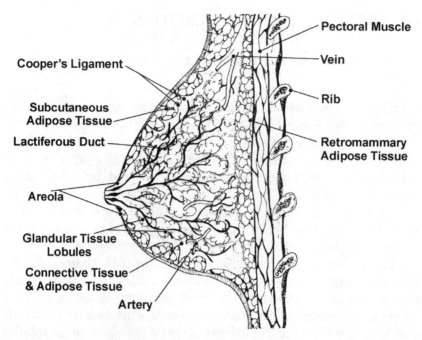

Figure 2.2   Lateral view of the female breast.

Source: Adapted with permission of the National Council on Radiation Protection and Measurements from NCRP Report No. 149, 2004.

consists of 20 or more lobes, which are each divided into numerous lobules (gland fields) each made up of 10 to 100 or more acini grouped around a collecting duct. The acini in the resting mammary gland are lined by a single layer of epithelial cells. An occasional second layer of epithelial cells around the base of the acinus is referred to as a myoepithelial cell layer. Myoepithelial cells of the breast resemble smooth muscle cells and take part in certain benign proliferations. The myoepithelial cells provide a muscular mechanism for ejecting milk from the acini and ducts. The bulk of the subareolar area and nipple is made of smooth muscle fibers—when the muscle fibers in the nipple contract, they empty the milk sinuses.

Microwave radiation in the Industrial, Scientific, Medical allocated band, from 902 to 928 MHz, is commonly used in clinical hyperthermia systems and is the primary frequency band considered here, especially 915 MHz, where MHz (megahertz) refers to 10^6 cycles per second. Microwave heating data of female breast tissues from a few published studies exist at 915 MHz, which is the desired operating frequency for the breast thermotherapy treatment described in this book; measured data suggest that carcinomas of the breast can be selectively heated compared to surrounding fatty breast tissues and glandular tissues.

Several articles with measured water content and other microwave-parameter data for breast tissues have been published by a number of authors, primarily Chaudhary et al,[36] Joines et al,[37] Surowiec et al,[38] Campbell and Land,[39] and Burdette.[40] The article by Burdette[40] provides measured microwave data for breast tissue at 500 MHz, 918 MHz, and 2450 MHz ($n = 3$ measurements per frequency); however, these data were measured through the skin and might not be completely representative of breast tissue itself (because of the effects of the skin on the measurements)—the 918-MHz measured dielectric constant was 38.0 and the ionic conductivity was 0.6 S/m; the 2.45-GHz measured dielectric constant was 32.0 and the ionic conductivity was 1.0 S/m. Note: The Campbell and Land article[**] has measured water content data and measured microwave dielectric properties data only for 3.2-GHz (gigahertz) microwaves.

As discussed in Section 2.1, the dielectric properties are usually quantified in terms of dielectric constant and electrical (ionic) conductivity, and they are quantified for normal breast tissue and breast cancer in **Figure 2.3** for 915-MHz microwaves. The relative dielectric constant primarily affects the wavelength of the microwaves propagating through tissue, and the electrical conductivity primarily affects the attenuation and power deposition of the microwaves in tissue. Increasing the dielectric constant of the tissue reduces the wavelength, and increasing the electrical conductivity increases the attenuation of microwaves. At 915 MHz, averaging the data from the Chaudhary ($n = 15$ measurements, 25°C) and Joines ($n = 12$ measurements, 24°C) articles, the average dielectric constant of normal breast tissue is 12.5, and the average ionic conductivity is 0.21 S/m. In contrast, for breast cancer tumors the average dielectric constant is 58.6 and the average ionic conductivity is 1.03 S/m. These values for normal breast tissue and breast cancer tumors are used later in Chapter 4 (Sections 4.3 and 4.6). Note: The data from the Chaudhary et al (C) and Joines et al (J) studies are measured at room temperature (24° or 25°C). It should be noted that as the temperature of tissue increases, generally the dielectric constant decreases

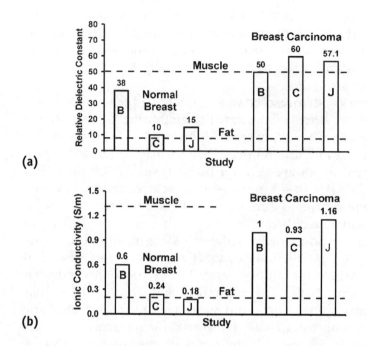

Figure 2.3   Measured dielectric parameters at approximately 915 MHz for normal breast tissue and breast carcinomas from three studies. B = Burdette,[40] C = Chaudhary,[36] J = Joines.[37] **(a)** Dielectric constant and **(b)** Ionic conductivity.

and the electrical conductivity increases. The dielectric parameters of normal breast tissues and breast cancer tumors are similar to low-water-content fatty tissue and high-water-content muscle tissue, respectively. It is further noted that normal breast tissue contains a mixture of fat, glandular, and connective tissues. Detailed microwave data of various tissues, including skin, muscle, and fat, are presented in an article by Gabriel et al.[41]

Table 2.1 summarizes the mean dielectric properties (dielectric constant, ionic conductivity, and microwave attenuation) of various tissues pertaining to the region of the breast. The microwave attenuation summarized in the last column of Table 2.1 is computed from the tissue dielectric constant and ionic conductivity according to equations given in Chapter 4 (Equations 4.5 and 4.8). Skin is high water content for which, at 915 MHz, the dielectric constant is equal to 50.0 and the ionic conductivity is 0.9 S/m (wet skin) and 0.6 S/m

Table 2.1 Estimated Mean Dielectric Parameters and Calculated
Microwave Attenuation for Tissues at 915 MHz Based
on Published Measured Data

Tissue Type	Dielectric Constant	Ionic Conductivity	Microwave Attenuation
Skin (wet)	50.0	0.9 S/m	2.1 dB/cm
Skin (dry)	50.0	0.6 S/m	1.4 dB/cm
Fat	8.0	0.08 S/m	0.5 dB/cm
Breast (normal)	12.5	0.21 S/m	1.0 dB/cm
Breast carcinoma	58.6	1.03 S/m	2.9 dB/cm
Benign tumor	50.0	1.0 S/m	2.3 dB/cm
Muscle	50.0	1.3 S/m	2.9 dB/cm
Blood	50.0	1.3 S/m	2.9 dB/cm
Bone	10.0	0.09 S/m	0.5 dB/cm
Lung (inflated)	20.0	0.4 S/m	1.4 dB/cm
Heart	50.0	1.3 S/m	2.9 dB/cm

Source: Data are based on Chaudhary et al[36]; Joines et al[37]; Gabriel et al[41].

S/m, Siemens per meter; dB/cm, decibels per centimeter.

(dry skin). Muscle and blood are high water content, and at 915 MHz they have a dielectric constant approximately equal to 50.0 and an ionic conductivity approximately equal to 1.3 S/m. Fat is low water content and has a dielectric constant equal to 8.0 and ionic conductivity equal to 0.08 S/m. Bone is low water content and has a dielectric constant equal to 10.0 and ionic conductivity equal to 0.09 S/m. Lung (inflated) has a dielectric constant equal to 20.0 and ionic conductivity equal to 0.4 S/m.

The article by Surowiec et al[38] has detailed measured data for selected glandular, ductal, fatty, and cancerous tissues in the frequency range 20 kHz (Kilohertz) to 100 MHz. Surowiec's measured data at low frequency indicate that breast tissue composed of normal connective tissue and normal glandular tissue has a significantly lower ionic conductivity compared to breast carcinomas, and the paper concludes that normal breast tissues are similar to adipose tissue. England and Sharples[42] at 9.4 GHz and England[43] at 3 GHz and 23.6 GHz measure dielectric parameter data for breast carcinoma. There does not appear to be any measured dielectric parameter data on pure ductal and glandular breast tissue for the frequency of interest, namely, 915 MHz.

A review article by Sha et al [44] comparing the results of published studies of the dielectric properties of normal and malignant breast tissue has recently been published. In Table 2.1, the dielectric parameters for breast carcinoma and normal breast are similar to muscle and fat, respectively. At 915 MHz, breast carcinoma has dielectric constant 58.6 similar to muscle, whereas normal breast has dielectric constant 12.5 similar to fat. At 915 MHz, the high ionic conductivity 1.03 S/m of breast carcinoma is similar to muscle, which has ionic conductivity 1.3 S/m, whereas normal breast tissue has dielectric constant 12.5 and ionic conductivity 0.21 S/m, which is closer to fat.

The article by Campbell and Land [39] provides measured dielectric parameter data at the microwave frequency of 3.2 GHz, and the percent water content for breast fat, glandular tissue, and connective tissue, benign tumors (including fibroadenomas), and malignant tumors. Note: In the Campbell and Land malignant tumor database, only 2 of 22 measurements were for samples frozen in liquid nitrogen and defrosted before measurements, which might affect the relative results for those two measurements. At 3.2 GHz, the Campbell and Land data show the following measured results for benign ($n = 18$ measurements) and malignant tumors ($n = 22$ measurements): the 3.2-GHz measured mean dielectric constant was 37.1 and 37.2 for benign and malignant tumors, respectively. The 3.2-GHz measured mean ionic conductivity was 2.2 S/m and 2.3 S/m for benign and malignant tumors, respectively. *Therefore, benign and malignant tumors are similar in their microwave properties and should heat equally when exposed to the same microwave electric-field amplitudes.*

Campbell and Land also report measured mean dielectric parameter data for breast fat and normal breast tissue (glandular and connective) at 3.2 GHz: the measured mean dielectric constant was 4.9 for breast fat and 25.3 for normal breast glandular and connective tissue; the mean ionic conductivity was 0.15 S/m for breast fat and 1.4 S/m for normal breast glandular and connective tissue. Campbell and Land's measured data of percent water content can also be used to assess the relative ability to heat breast tissues, that is, higher-water-content tissues heat faster than lower-water-content tissues do. From their values for measured water content (by weight) the following statistics for water content can be computed: breast fat ($n = 36$, range 11% to 31%, mean 19.1%, median 19.5%, 95% confidence interval 17.5% to 20.6%, standard deviation 4.6%), glandular and connective tissue ($n = 20$, range 41% to

76%, mean 58.4%, median 60.5%, 95% confidence interval 53.6% to 63.2%, standard deviation 10.4%), benign tumors including fibroad-rosis, fibrosis, and fibroadenoma ($n = 14$, range 60% to 84%, mean 71.6%, median 71.0%, 95% confidence interval 66.6% to 76.6%, standard deviation 8.6%), and malignant tumors ($n = 22$, range 66% to 79%, best values 75% to 80%, mean 74.3%, median 75.0%, 95% confidence interval 72.5% to 76.0%, standard deviation 4.0%). The mean and standard deviation values of water content for breast fat, glandular and connective tissue, breast carcinoma, and benign tumors are summarized graphically in **Figure 2.4**.

Based on a Mann-Whitney test, the median water content of normal breast glandular tissue (60.5%) and breast carcinoma (75.0%) differ significantly ($P < .0001$). Based on an unpaired t test with Welch correction, the mean water content of glandular tissue (58.4%) and benign lesions (71.6%) differs significantly (P = .0004). Thus, based on higher water content, it is expected that benign breast lesions and breast cancer tumors on average will heat significantly faster than glandular, connective, and fatty breast tissues will. A hypothesis that needs to be validated is that only the microscopic and visible tumor cells are preferentially heated with a 915-MHz microwave treatment, with all the surrounding fat, glandular, ductal, and connective tissues spared from significant heat damage because of lower water and lower ion content. Based on the similar water content of benign tumors

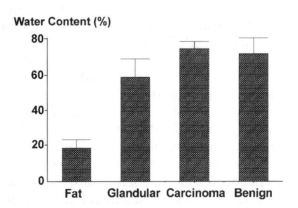

Figure 2.4　Measured water content (mean and standard deviation) for breast adipose tissue (fat), glandular and connective tissue, breast carcinoma, and benign tumors.[39]

(mean water content 71.6%) and malignant tumors (mean water content 74.3%), approximately equal heating would be expected when benign or malignant tumors are exposed to the same power level of microwave electromagnetic field.

As mentioned earlier, tissue electrical conductivity is a primary controlling parameter for tissue heating with microwave energy. Tissue electrical conductivity is also referred to as *tissue ionic conductivity* with units of S/m. Electrical conductivity is a function of the tissue properties, primarily the water content, ion content, and also the temperature of the tissue as described in a book by Duck.[45] The electrical conductivity increases as the water content, ion content, and temperature of the tissue increase.[46,47] For example, at 37°C, assuming 915-MHz microwaves, 0.9% physiological saline (9 g/kg) has a significantly higher (by a factor of 16) ionic conductivity (2.1 S/m) than pure water (0.13 S/m) does. Assuming 915-MHz microwaves, physiological saline at 37°C has a higher ionic conductivity (2.1 S/m) than room temperature (25°C) physiological saline (1.7 S/m) does.

Both tissue density and tissue specific heat have an inverse relation in regards to the microwave heating rate of tissue (refer to Equations 2.3 and 2.4). Based on measurements,[45] the mean value of breast fat density is 928 kg/m^3, normal breast is 1020 kg/m^3, and muscle is 1041 kg/m^3. I estimate that breast tumor density is similar to muscle. Based on measurements,[45] the specific heat of animal fat is approximately 2.5 Jg^{-1}K^{-1}, and the specific heat of animal muscle is approximately 3.7 Jg^{-1}K^{-1}. I assume that human breast fat and animal fat are similar in terms of specific heat, and I similarly assume that breast carcinoma and animal muscle have similar specific heat values. I estimate that the specific heat of normal breast tissue is on the order of 3.0 Jg^{-1}K^{-1}. Again, the difference (or ratio) in tissue electrical conductivity for normal breast (0.21 S/m) and breast carcinoma (1.03 S/m) is the primary preferential heating mechanism for 915 MHz microwaves. Using the above estimates for tissue properties (electrical conductivity, density, and specific heat), it can be shown (using Equations 2.3 and 2.4) that for a given value of electric field the thermal rise ratio for breast carcinoma compared to normal breast is approximately 3.0. That is, based on this simplified model represented by Equations 2.3 and 2.4, for a given value of 915 MHz microwave electric field, breast carcinomas should heat about three times faster than normal breast tissue (mixture of fat, glandular, ductal, and connective tissues).

Invasive or infiltrating breast cancer cells are often characterized as being moderately to poorly differentiated, meaning that they increasingly lose the ability to function as normal cells. As cancer cells lose their functionality, they can swell in size and absorb more water, thereby increasing the percent water content. Ions in a breast cancer cell play a significant role in the progression through the cell cycle as described by Ouadid-Ahidouch et al [48] and by Gallagher et al.[49] Ions are electrically charged particles, either positive or negative. The important ions in tissues include potassium (K^+), calcium (Ca^{2+}), sodium (Na^+), and chlorine (Cl^-). The calcium ion has two less electrons than protons and is positively charged $(2+)$. Calcium can attract and hold two chlorine (Cl^-) ions. Potassium can attract and hold only one chlorine (Cl^-) ion. The calcium and chloride ions in calcium chloride ($CaCl_2$) dissociate or separate and increase in mobility when dissolved in water, which increases the ionic conductivity of the water solution. Tightly clustered calcium deposits (known as microcalcifications) that appear on mammograms are often associated with carcinomas, another indication of the ions present in breast carcinomas. A tiny cluster of microcalcifications in a milk duct is usually attributed to precancer such as DCIS. Large chunks of calcium are usually associated with a benign lesion such as a fibroadenoma. Some of the calcifications appearing in the breast (but not associated with a breast lesion) are from calcium that leaves the bone, travels through the bloodstream, and then are randomly deposited within the breast.

Benign breast lesions are more common than cancerous lesions. Out of 1 million mammograms in which suspicious lesions are detected annually in the United States, approximately 800,000 will be categorized as benign and 200,000 will be proven cancerous based on pathology from biopsies. The breast tissue can contain one or more benign lesions, including cysts, fibroadenoma, benign fibrosis, benign fibroadrosis, benign epitheliosis, and papillomatosis. To quantify the relative heatability of benign tumors, in this section the ionic content and water content of benign lesions are described.

The ionic components in breast cyst fluid have been measured by Gairard et al[50] and by Bradlow et al.[51] Breast cyst fluids contain sodium (Na^+), potassium (K^+), calcium (Ca^{2+}), magnesium (Mg^{2+}), phosphate (PO_4^-), and chlorine (Cl^-) ions. Ions in breast cyst fluids having the highest mean concentrations are sodium (63.0 mEq/dL), potassium (91.2 mEq/dL), and chloride (56.6 mEq/dL) as depicted in **Figure 2.5** from Bradlow et al.[51] Bradlow et al cites three categories of breast cyst fluids:

- **Type I**: High concentration of potassium (K^+) compared to sodium (Na^+) and chloride (Cl^-)
- **Type II**: High concentrations of potassium (K^+) and sodium (Na^+) compared to chloride (Cl^-)
- **Type III**: High concentration of sodium (Na^+) compared to potassium (K^+) and chloride (Cl^-)

The high-ion contents of breast cysts should allow preferential heating of cysts with microwaves when compared to the heating of surrounding normal healthy breast tissue, which has lower ion contents. Therefore, during breast cancer ablation treatments with focused microwaves it might be possible that breast cysts in the surrounding tissues can also be ablated as a beneficial side effect.

Several types of cysts are described by Haagensen[52]: cystic disease is usually characterized by gross cysts 3 mm or larger accompanied by several benign microscopic cysts less than 3 mm in diameter. Microscopic cysts refer to nonpalpable tumors. Gross cysts (palpable tumors) include the following: (1) cysts containing inspissated

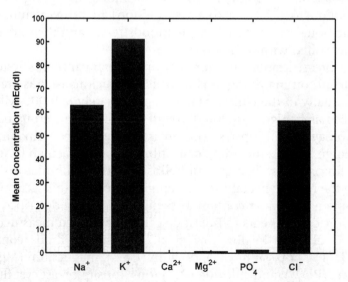

Figure 2.5   Measured mean concentrations of ions in breast cyst fluids.[51]

(thickened) milk—so-called galactoceles, (2) cysts evolving from duct ectasia, (3) cysts caused by fat necrosis, (4) cysts associated with intraductal papilloma—referred to as papillary cystadenoma, and (5) cysts induced by estrogen therapy.

Gross (very large) cysts can develop quickly and obtain a moderate persisting size, whereas some will decrease in size and in some cases disappear with time. A large percentage of gross cysts is discovered during the premenstrual or menstrual phase and enlarge rapidly, becoming painful and tender. Sometimes gross cysts are associated with signs of acute inflammation, pain, tenderness, and slight redness of the overlying skin. Once a needle aspiration procedure for removing the cyst fluid is performed, signs of inflammation rapidly subside. Gross cysts are most common in the age group between 30 and 54 years, or about 95% of cases. The more extensively the breast is examined, the greater the number of cysts is found.

Fibroadenomas (very common benign lesions, also called fibroids) are smooth and hard and can vary in size from 5 mm up to about 5 cm. Fibroadenomas have a high water content (mean 78.5%, $n = 6$) based on a small sample of measurements by Campbell and Land[39] and should be readily heated by microwave energy compared to surrounding healthy breast tissue. These benign lesions are usually clearly visible on mammography and ultrasound and can be surgically removed if desired. Some patients have multiple fibroadenomas, and breast-conserving surgery can become impractical for those patients—for those patients in particular, focused microwave thermotherapy might be have some benefit. Limited data exist for the measured water content of other benign tumors from the study by Campbell and Land as given as follows:

Benign fibrosis tumors: The median water content for one patient (age 26) in the Campbell and Land study was 65.5%, suggestive of high water content. *Fibrosis* refers to the formation of fibrous tissue that can occur as a reparative or reactive process. Fibrous breast disease is a special type of fibrosis that suppresses and obliterates both the acini of the lobules and the mammary ducts in a localized portion of the breast and that forms a palpable tumor. Fibrosis is abnormally firm, but not as hard as a carcinoma.

Benign fibroadrosis tumors: The median water content for one patient (age 27) in the Campbell and Land study was 73.5%, suggestive of high water content.

Benign epitheliosis (also known as papillomatosis) tumors: The median water content for one patient (age 40) in the Campbell and Land study was 61%, suggestive of high water content.

Benign adnosis tumors: The median water content for one patient (age 43) in the Campbell and Land study was 38%, suggestive of low water content. These tumors (benign adnosis) might not heat significantly compared to surrounding normal breast tissue, but only one data sample was measured and it might not be representative of other benign adnosis tumors.

In summary, benign lesions such as cysts, fibroadenomas, fibrosis, fibroadrosis, and epitheliosis (also known as papillomatosis) appear to be high water and high ionic content and should be readily heated and destroyed by microwave energy.

2.5 SUMMARY

This chapter has quantified the relative microwave thermal heating parameters for normal breast tissues, breast cancer, and benign breast lesions. Both breast cancer tumors and benign breast lesions tend to have high water and high ion contents, and when irradiated with microwave energy, they should heat more rapidly and to higher temperatures than the surrounding normal breast tissues that contain lower water content and lower ion content do. In the next two chapters, a detailed description of a clinical focused microwave thermotherapy system as well as the treatment methodology, theory, and analysis for focused microwave thermotherapy treatment of breast cancer are reviewed.

REFERENCES

1. Vernon CC, Hand JW, Field SB, et al. Radiotherapy with or without hyperthermia in the treatment of superficial localized breast cancer: results from five randomized controlled trials. *Int J Radiat Oncol Biol Phys.* 1996;35:731–744.
2. Valdagni R, Amichetti M. Report of long-term follow-up in a randomized trial comparing radiation therapy and radiation therapy plus hyperthermia to metastatic lymph nodes in stage IV head and neck patients. *Int J Radiat Oncol Biol Phys.* 1993;28:163–169.

3. Overgaard J, Gonzalez D, Hulshof MC, et al. Hyperthermia as an adjuvant to radiation therapy of recurrent or metastatic malignant melanoma. A multicentre randomized trial by the European Society for Hyperthermic Oncology. *Int J Hyperthermia.* 1996;12(1):3–20.

4. van der Zee J, Gonzalez D, van Rhoon GC, et al. Comparison of radiotherapy alone with radiotherapy plus hyperthermia in locally advanced pelvic tumors: a prospective, randomised, multicentre trial. *Lancet.* 2000;355:1119–1125.

5. Falk MH, Issels RD. Hyperthermia and oncology. *Int J Hyperthermia.* 2001;17(1):1–18.

6. Sugimachi K, Kuwano H, Ide H, Toge T, Saku M, Oshiumi Y. Chemotherapy combined with or without hyperthermia for patients with oesophageal carcinoma: a prospective randomized trial. *Int J Hyperthermia.* 1994;10(4):485–493.

7. Hall EJ. *Radiobiology for the Radiologist.* Philadelphia, Pa: JB Lippincott; 1994:262–263.

8. Perez CA, Brady LW. *Principles and Practice of Radiation Oncology.* 2nd ed. Philadelphia, Pa: JB Lippincott; 1992:396–397.

9. Streffer C. Hyperthermia and the therapy of malignant tumors. In: Streffer C, ed. *Cancer Therapy by Hyperthermia and Radiation.* New York: Springer-Verlag; 1987.

10. Bicher HI, Bruley DF. Hyperthermia. *Proceedings of the First Annual Meeting of the North American Hyperthermia Group;* August 23–25, 1981; Detroit, Michigan. New York, NY: Plenum Press; 1982.

11. Cheung AY, Samaras GM, eds. *J Microwave Power.* 1981;16(2)(special issue).

12. Hahn GM. *Hyperthermia and Cancer.* New York, NY: Plenum Press; 1982.

13. Lin JC, ed. *IEEE Trans on Microwave Theory and Techniques.* 1986;MTT-34(5)(special issue).

14. Steeves RA, Paliwal BR, eds. Syllabus: A categorical course in radiation therapy. *73rd Scientific Assembly and Annual Meeting of the Radiological Society of North America;* November 29–December 4, 1987; Oak Brook, Illinois.

15. Hill RP, Hunt JW. Hyperthermia. In: Tannock IF, Hill RP, eds. *Hyperthermia in the Basic Science of Oncology.* New York, NY: Pergamon Press; 1987:337–357.

16. Hinklebein W, Gruggmoser G, Engelhardt R, Wannenmacher M, eds. *Preclinical Hyperthermia. Recent Results in Cancer Research.* New York, NY: Springer-Verlag; 1988;109.

17. Steeves RA. Hyperthermia. *The Radiologic Clinics of North America.* Philadelphia, Pa: WB Saunders Company; 1989:27(3).

18. Sathiaseelan V, Mittal BB, Fenn AJ, Taflove A. In: Mittal BB, Purdy JA, Ang KK, eds. *Recent Advances in External Electromagnetic Hyperthermia. Advances in Radiation Therapy.* Norwell, MA: Kluwer Academic Publishers; 1998:213–245.

19. Lehmann JF, ed. *Therapeutic Heat and Cold.* 3rd ed. Baltimore, Md: Williams & Wilkins; 1982.

20. Coughlin CT. Clinical hyperthermic practice: interstitial heating. In: Field SB, Hand JW, eds. *An Introduction to the Practical Aspects of Clinical Hyperthermia.* London: Taylor & Francis; 1990:172–183.

21. Kapp DS, Meyer JL. Clinical hyperthermic practice: non-invasive heating. In: Field SB, Hand JW, eds. *An Introduction to the Practical Aspects of Clinical Hyperthermia.* London: Taylor & Francis; 1990:143–171.

22. Singletary SE. Minimally invasive techniques in breast cancer treatment. *Seminars in Surg Onc.* 2001;20:246–250.

23. Pfleiderer SO, Freesmeyer MG, Marx C, Kuhne-Heid R, Schneider A, Kaiser WA. Cryotherapy of breast cancer under ultrasound guidance: initial results and limitations. *Eur Radiol.* 2002;12:3009–3014.

24. Dowlatshashi K, Francescatti DS, Bloom KJ. Laser therapy for small breast cancers. *Am J Surg.* 2002;184:359–363.

25. Izzo F, Thomas R, Delrio P, et al. Radiofrequency ablation in patients with primary breast carcinoma. A pilot study of 26 patients. *Cancer.* 2001;92:2036–2044.

26. Huber PE, Jenne JW, Rastert R, et al. A new noninvasive approach in breast cancer therapy using magnetic resonance imaging–guided focused ultrasound surgery. *Cancer Res.* 2001;61:8441–8447.

27. Vargas HI, Dooley WC, Gardner RA, Gonzalez KD, Vanegas R, Heywang-Kobrunner SH, Fenn AJ. Focused microwave phased array thermotherapy for ablation of early-stage breast cancer: results of thermal dose escalation. *Ann Surg Oncol.* 2004;11(2):139–146.

28. Gerhard H, Klinger HG, Gabriel E. Short term hyperthermia: in vitro survival of different human cell lines after short exposure to extreme temperatures. In: Streffer C, ed. *Cancer Therapy by Hyperthermia and Radiation.* Baltimore, Md: Urban & Schwarzenberg; 1978:201–203.

29. Giovanella BC, Stehlin JS Jr, Morgan AC. Selective lethal effect of supranormal temperatures on human neoplastic cells. *Cancer Res.* 1976;36:3944–3950.

30. Bhowmick P, Coad JE, Bhowmick S, et al. *In vitro* assessment of the efficacy of thermal therapy in human benign prostatic hyperplasia. *Int J Hyperthermia.* 2004;20(4):421–439.

31. Sapareto SA, Dewey WC. Thermal dose determination in cancer therapy. *Int J Radiat Oncol Biol Phys.* 1984;10:787–800.

32. Durney CH. Electromagnetic field propagation and interaction with tissues. In: Field SB, Hand JW, eds. *An Introduction to the Practical Aspects of Clinical Hyperthermia.* London: Taylor & Francis; 1990:242–274.

33. National Council on Radiation Protection and Measurements. *A Guide to Mammography and Other Breast Imaging Procedures,* Bethesda, Md: National Council on Radiation Protection and Measurements; 2004:8. NCRP Report 149.

34. Love SM. *Dr. Susan Love's Breast Book.* 4th ed. Cambridge, Ma: Da Capo Press; 2005:202–212.

35. Haagensen CD. *Diseases of the Breast.* 3rd ed. Philadelphia, Pa: WB Saunders; 1986:8–46.

36. Chaudhary SS, Mishra RK, Swarup A, Thomas JM. Dielectric properties of normal and malignant human breast tissue at radiowave and microwave frequencies. *Indian J Biochem Biophys.* 1984;21:76–79.

37. Joines WT, Zhang Y, Li C, Jirtle RL. The measured electrical properties of normal and malignant human tissues from 50 to 900 MHz. *Med Phys.* 1994;21(4): 547–550.

38. Surowiec AJ, Stuchly SS, Barr JR, Swarup A. Dielectric properties of breast carcinoma and the surrounding tissues. *IEEE Trans Biomed Eng.* 1988:35(4):257–263.

39. Campbell AM, Land DV. Dielectric properties of female human breast tissue measured *in vitro* at 3.2 GHz. *Phys Med Biol.* 1992;37(1):193–210.

40. Burdette EC. Physical aspects of hyperthermia. In: Nussbaum GH, ed. *AAPM Medical Physics Monographs.* 1982;8:105–130.

41. Gabriel S, Lau RW, Gabriel C. The dielectric properties of biological tissues: Part III. Parametric models for the dielectric spectrum of tissues. *Phys Med Biol.* 1996;(41):2271–2293.

42. England TS, Sharples NA. Dielectric properties of the human body in the microwave region of the spectrum. *Nature.* March 26, 1949;163:477–488.

43. England TS. Dielectric properties of the human body for wave-lengths in the 1–10 cm range. *Nature.* September 16, 1950;166:480–481.

44. Sha L, Ward ER, Story B. A review of dielectric properties of normal and malignant breast tissue. *Proc IEEE SoutheastCon.* 2002:457–462.

45. Duck FA. *Physical Properties of Tissue.* New York, NY: Academic Press; 1990:167–223.

46. Stogryn A. Equations for calculating the dielectric constant of saline water. *IEEE Trans Microwave Theory and Techniques.* 1971;19(8):733–736.

47. Malmberg CG, Maryott AA. Dielectric constant of water from 0° to 100°C. *J Res National Bureau of Standards.* 1956;56(1):1–8.

48. Ouadid-Ahidouch H, Roudbaraki M, Ahidouch A, Delcourt P, Prevarskaya N. Cell-cycle-dependent expression of the large Ca^{2+}-activated K^+ channels in breast cancer. *Biochem Biophys Res Commun.* 2004;316:244–251.

49. Gallagher JD, Fay MJ, North WG, McCann FV. Ionic signals in T47D human breast cancer cells. *Cellular Signaling.* 1996;8(4):279–284.

50. Gairard B, Gros CM, Koehl C, Renaud R. Proteins and ionic components in breast cyst fluids. In: Angeli A, Bradlow HL, Dogliotti L, eds. *Endocrinology of Cystic Breast Disease.* New York, NY: Raven Press; 1983:191–195.

51. Bradlow HL, Skidmore FD, Schwartz MK, Fleisher M, Schwartz D. Cations in breast cyst fluid. In: Angeli A, Bradlow HL, Dogliotti L, eds. *Endocrinology of Cystic Breast Disease.* New York, NY: Raven Press; 1983:197–201.

52. Haagensen CD. *Diseases of the Breast.* 3rd ed. Philadelphia, Pa: WB Saunders; 1986:250–252.

Focused Microwave Thermotherapy for Treating Breast Cancer: System, Methodology, Theory, and Analysis

PART

II

Adaptive Focused Microwave Phased Array Thermotherapy System and Method for Treating the Intact Breast

3.1 INTRODUCTION

The previous chapter describes the detailed microwave properties of normal breast tissues and breast lesions. Microwave energy provides a means for selective heating of breast lesions compared to normal breast tissues, including breast fat and glandular tissues. At microwave frequencies, breast lesions are known theoretically to heat rapidly because of their high water and high ionic content. Unless special precautions are taken in the thermotherapy equipment design, skin is also high water content and could be readily heated and burned by microwaves delivered externally to the breast. An externally focused microwave thermotherapy system and treatment methodology for heating breast lesions within the intact breast without significantly heating and burning the skin is described in this chapter.

53

3.2 FOCUSED MICROWAVE ADAPTIVE PHASED ARRAY TECHNOLOGY AND BREAST THERMOTHERAPY TREATMENT METHODOLOGY

Focused microwave adaptive phased array technology has been used in radar systems over the last several decades.[1] In a typical microwave phased array radar application, focused microwave radiation is used to detect a target, for example, a missile as depicted in **Figure 3.1a**. In some radar problems, narrowband to ultrawideband jamming can interfere with the detection of the target, and, for that situation, an adaptive microwave phased array can be used to nullify automatically the microwave interference caused by the jamming either close to the radar or far away.[2,3] Adaptive microwave phased arrays can also be applied to cancer treatment in a similar fashion, and a theory applicable for narrowband to ultrawideband electromagnetic thermotherapy has been developed.[4] In applying adaptive phased arrays to general cancer treatment,[5] the tumor is the target and the skin and surrounding healthy tissues can be considered the regions where microwaves are to be nullified as shown in **Figure 3.1b**.

In the special case of breast cancer, to heat and kill breast cancer tumors or other lesions within the intact breast, in a novel treatment approach the breast is compressed, similar to mammography or stereotactic breast needle biopsy procedures, and two opposing microwave waveguide applicators external to the breast apply adaptively focused microwave energy,[6-10] as depicted in the artist's concept in Figure 1.5 and in the block diagram shown in **Figure 3.2**. To heat the breast tumor to a desired temperature, focused microwave phased array energy delivered to the two thermotherapy applicators is computer controlled during the treatment. The waveguide applicators[11] are typically spaced between 1 to 2 cm from the patient's skin and are designed to allow air cooling through the waveguide aperture. Air-cooled waveguide applicators have been used clinically in transcutaneous hyperthermia treatment of recurrent chest wall cancer and head and neck cancers, as described by Shidnia.[12] The air flowing through the thermotherapy applicator is affected by utilizing a perforated metal microwave-reflecting screen in the back wall of the applicator through which air is driven by a motorized fan system. An E-field feedback probe[13] at the central tumor depth d that measures the superimposed electric fields from the two waveguide applicators is

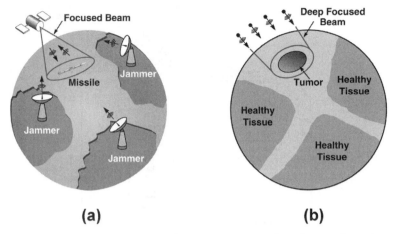

(a)   **(b)**

Figure 3.1   Comparison between adaptive microwave phased arrays for radar
application and for cancer treatment. (a) The adaptive radar uses
focused microwave radiation to detect a missile target while nullifying
jamming signals. (b) The adaptive microwave phased array thermotherapy system heats a cancerous tumor with focused microwave
radiation while nullifying any energy that might overheat surrounding healthy tissues.

Source: Chapple K. Deep focused heat kills tumors, leaves surrounding healthy tissue
unscathed. *Medical Equipment Designer*, April 2001, M14–M16.

used in focusing the microwaves with phase shifters in an adaptive
phased array.[7,8,14–16] A temperature probe in the target zone measures a
feedback signal and provides the measured data needed to adjust the
microwave power level to heat the tumor to a desired temperature.

Breast compression has a number of advantages for thermotherapy
treatments, compared to the situation when no compression is used.
Utilization of breast compression results in less penetration depth required to achieve microwave heating at central depth in tissue and reduces blood flow, which improves the ability to rapidly heat tumor
tissue. Compressing the breast to a flat surface with an acrylic plastic
material that is nearly transparent (introduces little attenuation) to microwaves[17] improves the transfer of microwave energy from the thermotherapy applicators to the breast tissue. Cooling the breast
compression plates and skin with air during thermotherapy treatments
helps reduce the potential for skin-surface hot spots. Compressing the
breast with the patient in a prone position (as depicted in **Figure 3.3**),
such as that used in stereotactic needle breast biopsy procedures,[18]
maximizes the amount of breast tissue within the compression device

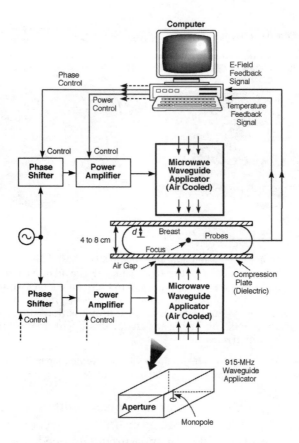

Figure 3.2   Block diagram for a focused microwave adaptive phased array thermotherapy system for heating a breast tumor in the compressed breast.

Source: Fenn AJ, Wolf GL, and Fogle RM. An adaptive microwave phased array for targeted heating of deep tumors in intact breast: animal study results. *Int J Hyperthermia* 1999;15(1):45–61. www.tandf.co.uk/journals Used with permission from Taylor & Francis.

and moves the breast lesion away from the chest wall. The prone patient orientation of the breast makes use of gravity to pull the breast tissue away from the chest wall.

Compression immobilizes the breast tissue such that any potential patient motion complications are eliminated. The plastic compression plate, which includes a rectangular aperture, allows ultrasound-imaging techniques to locate the tumor region accurately and to assist

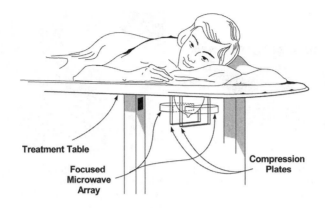

Treatment Table

Focused
Microwave
Array

Compression
Plates

Figure 3.3 Artist's depiction of a patient receiving focused microwave phased array thermotherapy. The patient is in prone position and the breast is compressed using plastic compression plates. Two opposing microwave thermotherapy applicators face the compressed breast.

Source: First published in US Patent Number 6,470,217, by A.J. Fenn, October 22, 2002 as Figure 6.

in the placement of the catheter required for the E-field focusing and temperature monitoring sensors. The amount of breast compression thickness can be varied from about 4 to 8 cm to accommodate patient tolerance during treatment. Ideally, for the most efficient tumor heating the two opposing microwave applicators should be positioned so that the tumor is in the center of the applicator aperture. Adequate tumor heating can be achieved, provided the tumor is located anywhere within the projected aperture of the applicators. It is estimated that 70% of patients have breast tumors that are located far enough from the chest wall and skin so that the tumor location falls within the aperture projected area, and these patients are potential candidates for this focused microwave phased array approach.

A Food and Drug Administration Investigational Device Exemption–approved two-channel 915-MHz focused microwave adaptive phased array thermotherapy system (developed by Celsion Corporation, Columbia, Maryland, under exclusive license from the Massachusetts Institute of Technology as the Microfocus-1000 APA Breast Thermotherapy System, now under exclusive license to Celsion [Canada] Limited, Ontario, Canada) was used in the clinical breast thermotherapy studies discussed in Chapters 6 through 9, as shown in **Figure 3.4**.

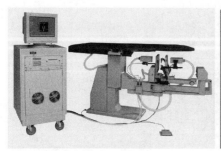

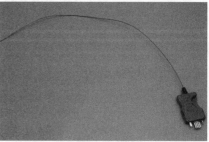

Figure 3.4 Focused microwave adaptive phased array thermotherapy system for treating breast cancer.

Source: Photo courtesy of Celsion (Canada) Limited.

Figure 3.5 Photograph of combination E-field and temperature probe for focused microwave thermotherapy treatments.

Source: Photo courtesy of Celsion (Canada) Limited.

This treatment system produces a focused microwave field in the breast to heat and destroy high-water-content, high-ion-content, malignant breast tumors, and microscopic carcinomas. A photograph of a combination E-field and temperature probe for use in a single catheter placed in the tumor during focused microwave thermotherapy treatments is shown in **Figure 3.5**. This combination E-field and temperature probe has an outer diameter equal to 1.1 mm and fits within a closed-end catheter. The temperature probe is at the tip and the E-field sensor is approximately 1.5 cm from the tip.

For thermotherapy treatment, the tumor is centrally located within the apertures of the compression plates, as depicted in **Figure 3.6**. After infiltrating a local anesthetic (1% lidocaine) at the desired entry point on the breast skin, the skin is nicked approximately 2.5 mm in length with an 11 blade and a catheter (flexible sharp closed-end plastic catheter, 1.65-mm [16-gauge] outer diameter, 1.22-mm inner diameter, Flexineedle, Best Industries, Springfield, Virginia) is inserted under ultrasound guidance, at the same depth d below the skin surface as the tumor tissue site in the breast. The catheter is inserted using one of two approaches: (1) A straight metal introducer (thin, rigid rod) is used to manually insert the sharp closed-end plastic catheter directly into the tumor bed under ultrasound guidance. The introducer provides the necessary mechanical stiffness to insert the flexible catheter through the breast tissue and into the tumor. (2) Another approach under ultrasound guidance is to use a needle biopsy gun to insert a hollow metal needle into the tumor, after which a long closed-end plastic catheter is inserted within the hollow metal needle, and then the needle is withdrawn leaving the closed-end plastic catheter in place—the length of the exposed plastic catheter can then be cut to the desired length. The combined E-field/temperature sensor (Figure 3.5) is then inserted to the tip of the catheter to measure the E-field (probe E in Figure 3.6) and temperature (probe 1 in Figure 3.6) in the tumor. Seven noninvasive temperature probes are attached to the skin surface (three on each compressed side of the breast), including one sensor at the nipple. Five of the skin sensors (2 to 6) are taped to the skin using sterile elastic skin closures or similar tape. Two of the skin sensors (7 and 8) can be located at or near the top of the compression plates and are in pressure contact with the chest wall skin region. It is generally desired that peak surface temperatures should not exceed approximately 41° to 42°C to avoid skin burns. To provide added protection against skin damage from the microwave fields, an air blower system with three or more flexible plastic tubes surrounding the breast provide additional airflow directed at the skin and nipple. For cases in which the breast is large, it might not be necessary to air cool the nipple, particularly if the tumor is located away from the nipple so that the nipple is out of the microwave field. Soft, thin pads are placed on the top edge of the compression plates so that there is less pressure on the skin when the patient is prone and the breast is in compression against the plates (**Figure 3.7**).

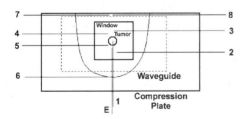

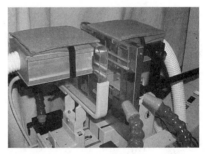

Figure 3.6 Diagram showing a projected view of the compressed breast with the projected aperture of the waveguide applicator and multiple probe (E-field and temperature) positions indicated.

Figure 3.7 Photograph showing the breast compression device, microwave applicators, cooling equipment, and cushion pads used in the focused microwave phased array breast thermotherapy treatments.

Source: Photo courtesy of Celsion (Canada) Limited.

The total thermal dose in the tumor is computer calculated and displayed on the computer system's monitor during the treatment. The treatment is completed and microwave power is turned off when the desired thermal dose is delivered to the tumor or the maximum treatment time (60 minutes) is reached. To determine the effectiveness of the treatment, pathology from needle core biopsy (single sample) and posttreatment lumpectomy tissue can be used to estimate tumor cell kill. Tumor cell kill based on tumor necrosis can be quantified from H and E pathology.

The total or cumulative equivalent minutes thermal dose is calculated from the measured temperatures recorded by the thermocouple sensors in the tumor. For example, in the Phase I focused microwave thermotherapy study, the desired tumor thermal dose during microwave heating was $CEM_{43°C} = 60$ minutes.[19] For thermal dose escalation investigation in the Phase II focused microwave thermotherapy study, the desired thermal dose during microwave heating was in the range of $CEM_{43°C} = 80$ to 120 minutes.[21,22] In these treatments, once the desired thermal dose is achieved, the microwave power is reduced to zero and there is a 5-minute cool-down period, with breast compression maintained. During this period, because of the thermal insulation of the surrounding breast tissues, the thermal dose might continue to accumulate in the tumor while the skin temperature rapidly drops to normal skin temperature values as a result of the surface air-cooling system.

3.3 REVIEW OF FOCUSED MICROWAVE BREAST THERMOTHERAPY TREATMENT PROCEDURES

Focused microwave breast thermotherapy, to date, is administered on an out-patient basis in an office-based setting in which the patient is fully awake during all of the procedures associated with the treatment. The patient receives a local anesthetic at the skin entry site for inserting one or two minimally invasive probes into the breast to monitor the treatment. The treatment parameters (microwave phase, microwave power, breast compression, and surface air cooling) are adjusted during the treatment to maintain patient comfort. In reference to **Figure 3.8**, the focused microwave breast thermotherapy treatment procedures are summarized as follows:

a. Catheter placement in breast tumor: Typically, one or two catheters with probes are inserted into the breast to monitor the microwave field and temperature in the tumor prior to and during treatment. Prior to inserting the catheter(s), a local anesthetic is infused at the skin entry point, and then the skin is nicked. Next, a closed-end plastic catheter (for a combined E-field/temperature sensor) is inserted under ultrasound guidance into the breast tumor. The appropriate catheter orientation is vertical once the patient is located in prone position— the patient can be either in prone or supine position during catheter insertion. Alternately, two separate catheters (one for E-field, one for temperature) are inserted in the breast, at two skin entry points, under ultrasound guidance into the breast tumor. To receive the vertically polarized microwave field properly, the E-field sensor catheter must be approximately vertical once the patient is located in prone treatment position, and to avoid microwave interference the temperature catheter must be horizontal if a metallic thermocouple sensor is used. If a fiber-optic temperature probe is used, it can be inserted at any angle in the breast and, generally, does not interfere with the focused microwaves.

b. Patient positioning on treatment bed and breast compression: The patient is positioned prone with the breast pendulant through a hole in the treatment table. The compression angle is adjusted to center the breast lesion within the central field or aperture of the applicators. The breast is compressed to a thickness of between about 4 and 8 cm (depending on the size of the breast and patient comfort) with the plastic compression plates. A compression thickness between about 4.5 and 6.5 cm is generally the most desirable.

c. Percutaneous probe sensor placement in catheter: The combined E-field/temperature sensor is inserted into the vertical plastic catheter until the tip of the sensor comes in contact with the closed end of the catheter. Alternately, separate E-field and temperature sensors are inserted into their respective catheters from part (a)—E-field vertical and temperature sensor horizontal.

d. Surface-temperature sensor placement: Five temperature probe sensors are attached to the skin surface (two on each side of the breast facing each of the two compression plates) and nipple (horizontal orientation) using thin sterile elastic skin closures or equivalent tape. Two additional temperature probes are placed in contact with the top of the compression plates (prior to breast compression) and the chest wall skin.

e. Microwave applicator placement: The two microwave applicators are positioned on opposite sides of the compression plates, with the lesion to be treated toward the midpoint of the applicator apertures, leaving an air gap of about 1.0 to 2.0 cm from the breast tissue to allow the desired airflow and surface cooling.

f. Microwave focusing: Under computer control, to focus the field at the E-field probe sensor position in the targeted breast tissue, the initial relative microwave phase delivered to each waveguide applicator is automatically determined.

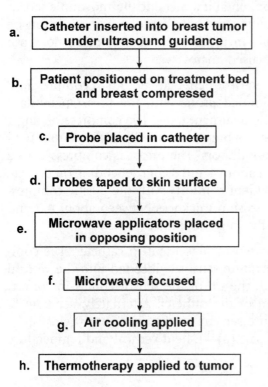

a. Catheter inserted into breast tumor under ultrasound guidance

b. Patient positioned on treatment bed and breast compressed

c. Probe placed in catheter

d. Probes taped to skin surface

e. Microwave applicators placed in opposing position

f. Microwaves focused

g. Air cooling applied

h. Thermotherapy applied to tumor

Figure 3.8

Flow diagram of focused microwave breast thermotherapy treatment procedure.

g. Surface air cooling: Once the desired phase setting for focusing the microwaves has been determined, the air-cooling system is enabled and airflow begins to cool the skin and nipple. The amount and direction of airflow from individual air tubes surrounding the breast are adjusted to cool the skin.

h. Begin focused microwave thermotherapy treatment: Once procedures (a) through (g) have been completed, the focused microwave treatment begins. The operator adjusts the absolute and relative microwave power of the two applicators during treatment to heat the tumor to both the desired target temperature and thermal dose, and to control the skin temperatures. The amount of breast compression is adjusted as necessary during treatment for patient comfort. The relative microwave phase delivered to the two microwave applicators is adjusted (refocused) during treatment to compensate for changes in the compression or positioning of the breast tissue, or to compensate for relative blood flow and thermal changes to tissue during treatment. The amount and direction of airflow from individual air tubes surrounding the breast to cool the skin are adjusted as needed during thermotherapy. The thermotherapy treatment is completed when a desired total thermal dose has been delivered by the microwave applicators, at which time the microwave power is turned off.

3.4 SUMMARY

This chapter has described focused microwave phased array technology and treatment methodology for thermotherapy treatment of breast cancer in the intact breast. The microwave phased array treatment system uses breast compression and opposing air-cooled microwave applicators along with a percutaneous microwave needle probe to focus microwave energy at a breast tumor mass, and temperature sensors are used to monitor the tumor temperature and surface temperatures. The next chapter describes the physics to understand and quantify the heating of breast lesions in the intact breast with focused microwave thermotherapy.

REFERENCES

1. Fenn AJ, Temme DH, Delaney WP, Courtney WE. The development of phased array radar technology. *Lincoln Laboratory Journal* (Massachusetts Institute of Technology). 2000;12(2):321–340.

2. Fenn AJ. Theory and analysis of near field adaptive nulling. *IEEE Antennas and Propagation Society International Symposium Digest.* June 8–13, 1986;2:579–582.

3. Fenn AJ. Evaluation of adaptive phased array antenna far-field nulling performance in the near-field region. *IEEE Trans Antennas and Propagation.* 1990;38(2):173–185.

4. Fenn AJ. *Application of Adaptive Nulling to Electromagnetic Hyperthermia for Improved Thermal Dose Distribution in Cancer Therapy.* Lexington, Mass: Massachusetts Institute of Technology, Lincoln Laboratory; July 3, 1991. Technical Report 917.

5. Fenn AJ. Adaptive hyperthermia for improved thermal dose distribution. In: Chapman JD, Dewey WC, Whitmore GF, eds. *Radiation Research: A Twentieth Century Perspective.* (Congress Abstracts). San Diego, Calif: Academic Press; 1991;1:290.

6. Fenn AJ. Minimally invasive monopole phased arrays for hyperthermia treatment of breast cancer. In: *Proceedings of the 1994 International Symposium on Antennas;* November 8–10, 1994; Nice, France; 418–421.

7. Fenn AJ. Minimally invasive monopole phased array hyperthermia applicators and method for treating breast carcinomas. US Patent Number 5,540,737. July 30, 1996.

8. Fenn AJ. Adaptive focusing and nulling hyperthermia annular and monopole phased array applicators. US Patent Number 5,441,532. August 15, 1995.

9. Fenn AJ, Wolf GL, Fogle RM. An adaptive microwave phased array for targeted heating of deep tumors in intact breast: animal study results. *Int J Hyperthermia.* 1999;15(1):45–61.

10. Gavrilov LR, Hand JW, Hopewell JW, Fenn AJ. Pre-clinical evaluation of a two-channel microwave hyperthermia system with adaptive phase control in a large animal. *Int J Hyperthermia.* 1999;15(6):495–507.

11. Cheung AY, Dao T, Robinson JE. Dual-beam TEM applicator for direct-contact heating of dielectrically encapsulated malignant mouse tumor. *Radio Science.* 1977;12(6(S)suppl):81–85.

12. Shidnia H, Hornback N, Ford G, Shen RN. Clinical experience with hyperthermia in conjunction with radiation therapy. *Oncology.* 1993;50:353–361.

13. Bassen H, Herchenroeder P, Cheung A, Neuder S. Evaluation of an implantable electric-field probe within finite simulated tissues. In: *Cancer Therapy by Hyperthermia and Radiation, Proceedings of the 2nd International Symposium.* Baltimore, Md: Urban & Schwarzenberg; 1978:15–25.

14. Fenn AJ, King GA. Adaptive radio-frequency hyperthermia-phased array system for improved cancer therapy: phantom target measurements. *Int J Hyperthermia.* 1994;10(2):189–208.

15. Fenn AJ, Sathiaseelan V, King GA, Stauffer PR. Improved localization of energy deposition in adaptive phased-array hyperthermia treatment of cancer. *J Oncol Management.* 1998;7(2):22–29.

16. Fenn AJ, King GA. Experimental investigation of an adaptive feedback algorithm for hot spot reduction in radio-frequency phased-array hyperthermia. *IEEE Trans Biomed Eng.* 1994;43(3):273–280.

17. von Hippel AR. *Dielectric Materials and Applications.* New York, NY: John Wiley and Sons; 1954:334.

18. Bassett L, Winchester DP, Caplan RB, et al. Stereotactic core-needle biopsy of the breast: a report of the Joint Task Force of the American College of Radiology, American College of Surgeons, and College of American Pathologists. *CA Cancer J Clin.* 1997;17:171–190.

19. Gardner RA, Vargas HI, Block JB, Vogel CL, Fenn AJ, Kuehl GV, Doval M. Focused microwave phased array thermotherapy for primary breast cancer. *Ann Surg Oncol.* 2002;9(4):326–332.

20. Vargas HI, Dooley WC, Gardner RA, Gonzalez KD, Venegas R, Heywang-Kobrunner SH, Fenn AJ. Focused microwave phased array thermotherapy for ablation of early-stage breast cancer: results of thermal dose escalation. *Ann Surg Oncol.* 2004;11(2):139–146.

21. Vargas HI, Dooley WC, Gardner RA, Gonzalez KD, Heywang-Kobrunner SH, Fenn AJ. Success of sentinel lymph node mapping after breast cancer ablation with focused microwave phased array thermotherapy. *Am J Surg.* 2003;186:330–332.

Focused Microwave Radiation Theory and Analysis

4.1 INTRODUCTION

This chapter reviews the necessary physics for understanding and quantifying the transcutaneous delivery of focused microwave phased array energy to breast tissues, including breast tumors. Background on the generation of microwaves and the addition of microwaves from multiple coherent antenna radiators (also known as a *phased array antenna*) are discussed in Section 4.2. Section 4.3 describes a simplified theory and analysis for microwave energy propagating through tissue. The concepts of microwave energy dose and tissue thermal dose and their computation are reviewed in Sections 4.4 and 4.5, respectively. A more detailed electromagnetic simulation of a focused microwave phased array thermotherapy system for treatment of breast cancer is then described in Section 4.6.

4.2 GENERATION AND ADDITION OF MICROWAVE FIELDS

Consider **Figure 4.1**, which depicts the basic problem of generating microwave energy that is to be aimed in the direction of tissue containing tumor to be treated. A required component in a microwave thermotherapy system is a microwave oscillator that produces a continuous wave (CW) voltage oscillating sinusoidally at a desired microwave frequency, say, 915 megahertz (MHz), as commonly used in thermotherapy. The output of the microwave oscillator is directed, by means of a coaxial cable, into an electronically controlled microwave amplifier that increases the microwave average CW power to an adjustable desired level typically in the range of 0 to 100 watts (W) for thermotherapy treatments. The power-amplified 915-MHz microwave energy is then directed by means of another coaxial cable to a wire probe antenna (formed by extending the center conductor of the coaxial cable) inside a metal waveguide structure that aims the microwave energy at the target tissue. The voltage oscillating at the junction of the wire probe antenna and outer conductor of the coaxial cable creates an acceleration of electric charges on the metallic wire, which in turn produces an oscillating electric current, denoted $i(t)$ (where i is the current and t is time) flowing through the wire.

The sinusoidally oscillating electric current flowing through the wire probe antenna generates a time-varying (sinusoidal) electromagnetic field that propagates inside the metal waveguide. The electromagnetic field, with electric and magnetic field components,

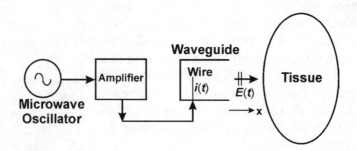

Figure 4.1   Generation and radiation of microwave energy for thermotherapy treatments.

propagates away from the wire probe antenna within the waveguide, and then is emitted as microwave radiation (photons) from the open end of the waveguide toward the tissue.

The generated instantaneous microwave electric field $E(t)$ that irradiates the tissue will oscillate sinusoidally[1] at the same frequency (f) as the microwave oscillator. The microwave electric field will be polarized primarily in the same direction as the wire probe orientation in the waveguide, for example a vertically oriented wire probe produces a microwave field that is primarily vertically polarized. The propagation of the electromagnetic wave energy through the coaxial cables, waveguide, air, and tissue is governed by Maxwell's equations.[1] In the following paragraphs, the propagation and addition of opposing plane-wave microwave fields are described quantitatively.

The instantaneous sinusoidal oscillation of a plane-wave electric field propagating in the positive x direction through free-space vacuum is represented mathematically in general by

$$E_p(t,x) = \sin(\omega t - \beta(x - x_p) - \phi_p(t)) \tag{4.1a}$$

or for a similar plane-wave electric field propagating in the negative x direction by

$$E_n(t,x) = \sin(\omega t + \beta(x - x_n) - \phi_n(t)) \tag{4.1b}$$

where $\sin(\ )$ is the trigonometric function, $\omega = 2\pi f$ is the radian frequency, $\beta = 2\pi \div \lambda$ is the propagation constant, λ (lambda) is the wavelength of the microwave radiation, x_p and x_n are arbitrary spatial displacements for the plane waves (providing fixed phase offsets relative to the effective origin of the plane-wave radiation), and $\phi_p(t)$ and $\phi_n(t)$ are arbitrary phase shifts that can be controlled by individual phase-shifting devices as a function of time (t). Ignoring any tissue properties for the moment, Equations 4.1a and 4.1b can be simply viewed as representing ideal plane-wave electric fields from opposing microwave applicators located at positions x_p and x_n that surround a focal point in space at $x = 0$. Because only the relative phase between the two electric fields is of importance in focusing, for convenience, let $\phi_p = 0$ and $\phi_p = \phi(t)$. Note: The quantity $\phi(t)$ can be viewed as the adaptive phase shift produced by an electronically controlled phase-shifting device used in focusing the microwave radiation when two opposing microwave applicators are used to irradiate a tumor in tissue. Now, let

$$\Phi(t,x) = \omega t - \beta x - \phi(t) \tag{4.2}$$

represent the overall or total phase angle of the microwave radiation as a function of time t, position x, and time-dependent phase shift $\phi(t)$. For convenience, assume a fixed position $x = 0$ and no time-varying additional phase shift $\phi(t) = 0$ so that $\Phi = \omega t$. As time increases, the phase angle increases linearly as ωt.

Two full cycles of the electric-field amplitude $E(t) = \sin(\Phi) = \sin(\omega t)$ are depicted in **Figure 4.2** in which a complete amplitude oscillation occurs for every 360 degrees of phase variation. In this example, the following relation between phase Φ, frequency f, and time t applies:

$$\Phi = 360° \, ft \tag{4.3}$$

Thus, for $f = 915$ MHz, 360 degrees of phase variation of the microwave field occur in a time period of $t = 1 \div f = 1.093$ nanoseconds (1.093×10^{-9} seconds).

It should be noted that the microwave oscillating frequency 915 MHz is attractive for breast thermotherapy treatments for a number of reasons:

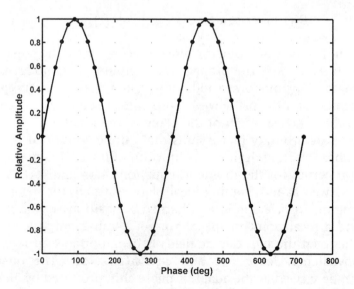

Figure 4.2   Sinusoidal variation of the electric field as a function of phase.

1. 915-MHz microwave radiation rapidly heats high-water-, high-ion-content breast cancer tumors and benign breast lesions compared to the surrounding normal breast tissue.

2. 915-MHz microwave radiation propagates with an attenuation of about 1 dB/cm in normal breast tissue; thus, a significant portion of the microwave energy can reach a breast tumor at central depth when opposing phase-coherent microwave applicators are used in a focused manner.

3. The 9-cm wavelength of 915-MHz microwave radiation in breast tissue is favorable for focusing energy at a central depth in the breast with two microwave applicators opposing the breast, and because of interference between the two opposing waves a reduced microwave field simultaneously occurs at each of the opposing skin surfaces.

4. Required microwave components such as power amplifiers (to generate the desired amount of power deposition) and phase shifters (to control the timing and focusing of the two microwave fields radiating from the two applicators) are readily available at 915 MHz.

5. Noncontact air-cooled applicators for delivering focused 915-MHz microwave treatments with a large heating field for treating a large volume of breast tissue while cooling the skin have been developed.

6. 915 MHz is an approved radiating frequency in the Industrial, Scientific, and Medical band; therefore, a shielded room is generally not required for focused microwave thermotherapy treatments.

Conceptually, as depicted in **Figure 4.3**, if only a *single external* (transcutaneous) microwave applicator irradiates tissue, for frequencies above about 300 MHz much of the microwave energy is absorbed in the superficial tissue layers and little energy is deposited in the deep tumor.[2] The absorbed microwave energy in tissue produces molecular friction (as a result of ion motion in reaction to the oscillating microwave field) and heat, which elevates the tissue temperature. The magnitude of the molecular friction and heat is proportional to the specific absorption rate (SAR) of the tissue as described quantitatively in the sections that follow. The fundamental problem in heating deep tumors with externally applied microwave energy is to avoid heating and burning the superficial tissues. Focused microwave arrays, using electrical phasing, have been considered for deep heating of tumors as first described in a 1973 research report by von Hippel.[3] The ability to focus microwave energy on a tumor relies heavily on implementing the proper phase relation between two or more microwave applicators. An adaptive phased array thermotherapy system is a new approach for reliably heating deep tumors.[4-6] As depicted in **Figure 4.4**, two microwave phased array applicators surround the tissue containing the tumor to be heated. A microwave sensor probe in the tumor is used as feedback in a computer-controlled system to adaptively adjust the timing of the microwave radiation electric fields, denoted E_1 and E_2, from applicators 1 and 2, respectively. In this adaptive phased array treatment system, the total microwave field and SAR in the deep tumor is significantly enhanced while limiting the intensity of the microwave field in the superficial tissues.

The contrast between unfocused and focused microwaves is now quantified by an example with a geometry similar to Figure 4.4, but

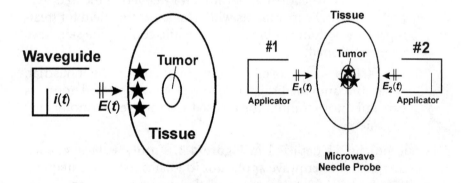

Figure 4.3 Artist's depiction of a single external microwave applicator for superficial tissue treatment. Most of the microwave energy emitted from the applicator is absorbed (represented qualitatively by the location of star symbols) in the superficial layers creating high superficial temperatures before the deep tissue can be heated.

Figure 4.4 Artist's depiction of two focused microwave phased array applicators surrounding tissue containing a centrally located tumor. The star symbols are intended to be qualitative and represent the location of the peak elevated temperature region at the tumor.

ignoring (for the moment) any tissue effects. For a simplified case of opposing plane waves as expressed by Equations 4.1a and 4.1b surrounding a desired focal point at $x = 0$, let the reference positions be defined by $x_p = \lambda$ and $x_n = -\lambda$ (that is, for convenience the plane wave reference positions are displaced one wavelength on either side of the focal point). Assume that the unfocused microwave example corresponds to an out-of-phase situation where $\phi_p(t) = 135°$ and $\phi_n(t) = 0°$, and the focused microwave example corresponds to the in-phase condition $\phi_p(t) = \phi_n(t) = 0°$. Next, these phase values can be substituted into Equations 4.1a and 4.1b, and the 915-MHz electric-field amplitude can be computed over two periods of oscillation (equivalent time period of 2.186 nanoseconds). **Figure 4.5** depicts the unfocused and focused microwave examples in which two microwaves with unity amplitude incident at the focal point are either constantly out of phase by a relative phase shift of $\phi(t) = 135°$ or they are constantly in phase $\phi(t) = 0°$. The effective microwave power, denoted $P(t)$, is proportional to the square of the total microwave electric-field magnitude, that is, $P(t) = C|E_1(t) + E_2(t)|^2$, where C is a constant. When the two microwave fields are unfocused, there is a substantial timing error or phase-shift error such that the electric fields ($E_1(t)$, $E_2(t)$) do not add up significantly in the tumor. If the two microwave electric fields are in accurate time alignment, the two oscillating electric fields add together significantly and the microwave power density is amplified continuously in the tumor. If $E_1(t) = E_1(t)$), then $P(t) = 4C|E_1(t)|^2$. If one of the fields is zero, say $E_2(t) = 0$, then $P(t) = C|E_1(t)|^2$. Therefore, the focal power of a coherent focused array is a factor of four times the power when a single applicator is radiating.

4.3 SIMPLIFIED THEORY AND ANALYSIS FOR MICROWAVE PROPAGATION IN TISSUE

Microwave energy from a thermotherapy applicator radiates into tissue typically as a spherical wave with the electric-field amplitude varying, in part, as the inverse of the distance x from the applicator (refer to Figure 4.3). There will be a partial reflection[1] of the microwave energy once the microwaves encounter the air/tissue boundary.

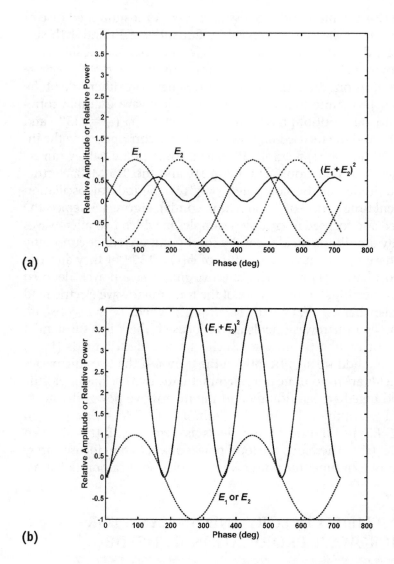

Figure 4.5   Example quantitative comparison of the addition of unfocused versus focused microwaves at a point in space. **(a)** Unfocused microwaves in which the two microwaves have the same oscillating frequency but are 135 degrees out of phase and the resulting total microwave power is low. **(b)** Focused microwaves in which the two microwaves have the same oscillating frequency and are in phase and the resulting total microwave power is high.

Additionally, once the spherical wave enters the tissue, the microwave field amplitude decays as an exponential function of the product of the attenuation constant α of the body tissue and the distance d traversed (or depth) within the body. The microwave electric-field phase varies linearly with distance according to the product of the phase propagation constant β in tissue and distance d. For simplicity, a coherent (phase-synchronized) phased array of dual-opposing breast thermotherapy applicators is analyzed here under the assumption that the applicator radiation can be approximated by a plane wave (characterized by a flat wave front). Mathematically, ignoring the sinusoidal time variation (which carries through all subsequent field expressions), the plane-wave electric field amplitude versus depth, denoted $E(d)$, in tissue is given simply by

$$E(d) = E_0 \exp(-\alpha d) \exp(-i\beta d) \tag{4.4}$$

where E_0 is the surface electric field (in general represented by an amplitude and phase angle), *exp* is the exponential function, and i is the imaginary number (Gauthrie)[7].

For homogeneous dielectric media (also referred to as conducting media) with permittivity ϵ, permeability μ, and electrical conductivity σ, the attenuation and phase constants at radian frequency $\omega = 2\pi f$, where f is the frequency, are calculated as

$$\alpha = \omega\sqrt{\mu\epsilon}\left\{\frac{1}{2}\left[\sqrt{1+\left(\frac{\sigma}{\omega\epsilon}\right)^2}-1\right]\right\}^{\frac{1}{2}} \tag{4.5}$$

$$\beta = \omega\sqrt{\mu\epsilon}\left\{\frac{1}{2}\left[\sqrt{1+\left(\frac{\sigma}{\omega\epsilon}\right)^2}+1\right]\right\}^{\frac{1}{2}} \tag{4.6}$$

where $\epsilon = \epsilon_r \epsilon_0$ with ϵ_r the relative real dielectric constant, $\epsilon_0 = 8.854 \times 10^{-12}$ F/m is the permittivity of free space, and $\mu = \mu_0 = 1.257 \times 10^{-6}$ H/m is the permeability of free space. The wavelength of the dielectric medium is calculated as

$$\lambda = \frac{2\pi}{\beta} \tag{4.7}$$

The relative field attenuation A as a function of distance d into tissue, or transmission loss of a plane wave in decibels per meter (dB/m), can be calculated by

$$A(d) = 20 \log_{10}(\exp(-\alpha d)) \tag{4.8}$$

As discussed later, plane-wave electromagnetic energy, at the microwave frequency 915 MHz, attenuates at a rate of about 3 decibels (3 dB or one-half power) per cm in high-water-, high-ion-content tissues, such as breast tumor or muscle, and about 1 dB per cm in normal glandular and fatty breast tissue. Thus, a single radiating applicator has a significant fraction of its microwave energy absorbed by intervening superficial body tissue compared to the energy that irradiates deep tissue, likely creating a hot spot in superficial tissue. Because skin surface cooling with either air or water protects tissue only to a maximum depth of about 0.25 cm, to avoid hot spots it is necessary to introduce a second phase-coherent applicator that has the same microwave radiation amplitude as the first applicator. The second phase-coherent CW applicator can theoretically increase the average power (and hence the energy) delivered to deep tissue by a factor of four compared to a single applicator, as shown in section 4.2 and described by Field and Hand.[8]

The phase characteristics of the electromagnetic radiation from two or more applicators (known as a phased array) can have a pronounced effect on the distribution of power delivered to different tissues. From Equation 2.3, the relative SAR in homogeneous tissue (no variation in tissue conductivity or density, for example) is simply equal to the square of the electric-field amplitude, that is:

$$SAR_{homogeneous} = |E|^2 \tag{4.9}$$

A simplified case, homogeneous breast tissue, in which the microwave radiation is focused at a central tissue site is described in detail here. In a simplified analysis,[9] ray tracing can be used to analyze breast phantom tissue irradiated by dual opposing microwave phased array applicators.

From Equations 4.5 and 4.6, at 915 MHz for homogeneous normal breast tissue (with approximate dielectric constant 12.5 and electrical conductivity 0.21 S/m [Siemens per meter; values averaged from Chaudhary et al[10] and Joines et al[11]]), the calculated attenuation constant α is 0.11 radians/cm and the phase propagation constant β is 0.69 radians/cm, or 39.5 electrical degrees per cm. It follows from Equation 4.7 that the wavelength in normal breast tissue is approximately 9.0 cm at 915 MHz, and from Equation 4.8 the microwave loss is calculated to be approximately 1 dB/cm.

A typical range of breast tissue thickness for focused microwave thermotherapy treatments varies from about 4.0 cm to 8.0 cm. For a breast phantom thickness of, say, 4.5 cm the electric field of a single applicator radiating on the left side is E_0 at the surface, $-i\,0.8E_0$ (where the pure imaginary component represents a 90-degree phase shift) at the central position (2.25 cm deep), and $-0.6E_0$ at the right surface with the negative sign representing a 180-degree phase shift. Therefore, the two waves are completely out of phase on the phantom surface and will partially cancel because the amplitudes are unequal. Combining the microwave radiation from the two phase-coherent applicators yields an electric-field value of $0.4E_0$ on both surfaces (from Equation 4.9, $SAR = 0.16E_0^2$) and $-i\,1.6E_0$ at the central position (2.25 cm depth) ($SAR = 2.56E_0^2$). Thus, for phantom breast tissue with 4.5-cm thickness and opposing focused applicators, there is a significantly lower SAR at the surface, by a factor of 16 compared to the central SAR.

As a second example, for a breast phantom thickness of, say, 6.0 cm the magnitude of the electric field of a single applicator radiating on the left side is E_0 at the surface, $0.707E_0$ at the central position (3.0 cm deep), and $0.5E_0$ at the right surface. The phase shift for a 915-MHz electromagnetic wave (9-cm wavelength in breast) passing through 6 cm of breast tissue will be $\beta d = 360° \times 6 \text{ cm} \div 9 \text{ cm} = 240°$. Therefore, the two waves are partly out of phase on both the right and left sides of the breast phantom surfaces and will partially cancel because the phases are not equal. Combining the microwave radiation from the two phase-coherent applicators yields an electric-field value of $0.75E_0$ on both surfaces and $2E_0$ at the central position (3.0 cm depth). Thus, for a 6-cm-thick breast phantom and opposing focused microwave applicators, there is a significantly lower SAR at the surface, by a factor of 7.1, compared to the central SAR.

Now, assume a more general case for a 6-cm-thick breast phantom in which the opposing microwave applicators are not necessarily phase aligned. Assume applicator 1 on the left side of the breast has a constant 0-degree phase, and applicator 2 on the right side of the breast has a variable phase shift ϕ_2. The electric field measured by an E-field probe at the central focus (in the tumor) is simply the coherent combination of the fields from the two applicators:

$$E_{focus} = 0.707 + 0.707(\cos\phi_2 + i\sin\phi_2) =$$
$$0.707(1 + \cos\phi_2) + i\,0.707\sin\phi_2 \qquad (4.10)$$

The power (or SAR) at the focus is equal to the square of the magnitude of the focal electric field given by Equation 4.10, or

$$SAR_{focus} = 0.5(1 + \cos\phi_2)^2 + 0.5\sin^2\phi_2 \qquad (4.11)$$

Now assume a 6-cm breast thickness so that in the breast tissue $\beta d = 240°$. Then, the electric field (E) and SAR at each skin surface can be expressed as

$$E_{Left\ Skin} = 1 + 0.5(\cos(\phi_2 - 240°) - i\sin(\phi_2 - 240°)) \qquad (4.12)$$

$$SAR_{Left\ Skin} = (1 + 0.5(\cos(\phi_2 - 240°))^2$$
$$+ (0.5\sin(\phi_2 - 240°))^2 \qquad (4.13)$$

$$E_{Right\ Skin} = [\cos\phi_2 + i\sin\phi_2] + [0.5\cos(-240°)$$
$$+ 0.5\,i\sin(-240°)] \qquad (4.14)$$

$$SAR_{Right\ Skin} = (\cos\phi_2 + 0.5\cos(240°))^2$$
$$+ (\sin\phi_2 - 0.5\sin(240°))^2 \qquad (4.15)$$

Again, assuming 6-cm breast tissue thickness, using Equations 4.11, 4.13, and 4.15, **Figure 4.6** shows the SAR on the left and right skin surfaces and in the central tissue site (tumor) as the relative phase shift of Channel 2 (ϕ_2) varies from -180 degrees to $+180$ degrees. In the central tissue site (tumor), a single peak occurs when the phase of Channel 2 is $0°$, and a null occurs when the phase is either plus or minus $180°$. A reduced value of SAR occurs on both skin surfaces when the phase is $0°$, that is, the array is focused. In practice, the phase focusing is accomplished by means of an E-field sensing probe in the tumor, an adaptive phased array control algorithm, and an electronic circuit network that adjusts the phase relation between the microwave applicators.

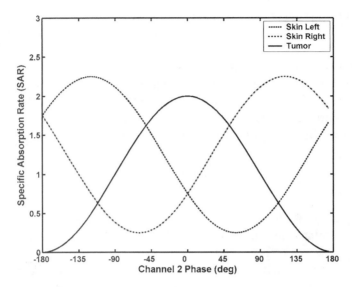

Figure 4.6   Calculated specific absorption rate (SAR) in simulated 6-cm thick homogeneous breast tissue at the left and right skin surfaces and in the central tumor position as a function of relative phase shift between the two opposing applicators.

The adaptive phased array breast treatment system uses two microwave channels, fed by a common oscillator, containing two electronically adjustable phase shifters to focus the microwave energy at an E-field feedback probe. This adaptive phased array system has significant advantage over a nonadaptive phased array. A nonadaptive phased array with two channels could, in theory, produce a null, a maximum, or an intermediate value of E-field depending on whether the two waves are 180 degrees out-of-phase, completely in-phase, or partly out-of-phase, respectively. That is, the microwave phase delivered to the microwave applicators can be adjusted between –180 degrees and 180 degrees before and during the treatment to create and maintain a focused field in the breast tissue. The phase shift experienced by the microwave field transmitted through breast tissue partly cancels or nulls the opposing field entering the tissue. Because of destructive interference of the microwaves away from the central focus, lower temperatures in the superficial breast tissues would be expected.

Because the adaptive phased array automatically focuses the E-field in the presence of all scattering structures in the tissue, this type of array should provide reliable deep focused heating.

4.4 CALCULATION OF MICROWAVE ENERGY DOSE

Electrical energy consumption is commonly expressed in units of kilowatt-hours. For example, a 100-W light bulb operating for 10 hours consumes 1 kilowatt-hour of electrical energy. Mathematically, the time-dependent expression for the microwave energy dose W delivered by a thermotherapy applicator is given by (refer to Vitrogan[12]):

$$W = \Delta t \sum_{i=1}^{N} P_i \qquad (4.16)$$

In Equation 4.16, Δt represents the constant intervals (in seconds) in which microwave power is measured, and the summation, denoted $\sum$, is computed over N time samples during the complete treatment period with the power (in watts) in the ith interval denoted by P_i. In Equation 4.16, the energy can refer to the commanded microwave energy or the net energy transferred to tissue taking account of any reflected energy from the tissue.

In thermotherapy treatments, the microwave energy W has units of watt-seconds, which is also designated as joules. The units of kilojoules (1000 joules) are also commonly used in which 1 kJ = 1 kW-s. For example, in a simplified focused microwave treatment depicted in **Figure 4.7**, each of two channels could supply 50 watts for 5 minutes (300 seconds), and then the power is increased to 60 watts for 15 minutes (900 seconds). For this example, the total microwave energy dose delivered in 20 minutes (1200 seconds) is calculated as:

$$
\begin{aligned}
W &= 2\,((50 \text{ watts} \times 300 \text{ seconds}) \\
&\quad + (60 \text{ watts} \times 900 \text{ seconds})) \\
&= 138,000 \text{ watt-seconds} \\
&= 138,000 \text{ joules} \\
&= 138.0 \text{ kJ} \qquad (4.17)
\end{aligned}
$$

In clinical treatments, the microwave power level of each of the two channels is adjusted as needed in raising the tumor to the target temperature and equivalent thermal dose while keeping the skin temperatures at safe levels.

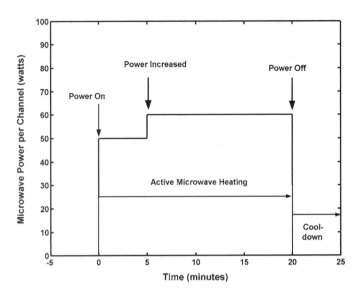

Figure 4.7 Simplified example of a focused microwave treatment in which the microwave power of each of two treatment channels is 50 watts (100 W total) for the first 5 minutes and then is raised to 60 watts per channel (120 W total) for the remaining 15 minutes of treatment. The total microwave energy dose is calculated to be 138 kilowatt-seconds or equivalently 138 kilojoules.

4.5 CALCULATION OF EQUIVALENT THERMAL DOSE

As described by Sapareto and Dewey,[13] the cumulative or total equivalent thermal dose relative to 43°C (CEM$_{43°C}$) is calculated as a summation:

$$\text{CEM}_{43°C} = \Delta t \sum_{i=1}^{N} R^{(43-T_i)} \tag{4.18}$$

where the symbol $\sum$ in Equation 4.18 represents the summation over a series of temperature measurements during the treatment, T_i is the series of temperature measurements ($T_1, T_2, T_3, \ldots, T_N$), Δt is the constant interval of time (units of minutes, usually a fraction of a minute) between measurements, R is a rate that is equal to

0.5 if $T > 43\,^{\circ}$C and R is equal to 0.25 if $T < 43\,^{\circ}$C. The cumulative equivalent minutes ($CEM_{43^{\circ}C}$) thermal dose calculation is useful for assessing any possible heat damage to the breast tumor, skin, and other tissues.

Equation 4.18 is an empirical model developed by Sapareto and Dewey based on in vitro and in vivo cell survival data, and the use of $43\,^{\circ}$C for the reference temperature is a best estimate for when thermotherapy begins to cause a significantly faster rate of cancer cell kill. In the case of multiple thermotherapy treatments, the overall cumulative thermal dose is defined as being equal to the summation of the cumulative thermal dose achieved in each treatment (see, for example, Jones[14]). Using Equation 4.18, **Table 4.1** gives the relation between treatment temperature (in the range of $40\,^{\circ}$ to $53\,^{\circ}$C for a constant 1-minute treatment time) and equivalent thermal dose.

Table 4.1   Calculated Equivalent Thermal Dose Factor for 1 Minute of Heating as the Temperature Varies from $40\,^{\circ}$ to $53\,^{\circ}$C Using the Sapareto and Dewey Model

Temperature (°C)	Difference (43° − T)	Exponential Factor $R^{(43°-T)}$	Equivalent Thermal Dose Factor (minutes/minute)
40	−3	4^{-3}	0.0156
41	−2	4^{-2}	0.0625
42	−1	4^{-1}	0.250
43	0	2^{0}	1
44	1	2^{1}	2
45	2	2^{2}	4
46	3	2^{3}	8
47	4	2^{4}	16
48	5	2^{5}	32
49	6	2^{6}	64
50	7	2^{7}	128
51	8	2^{8}	256
52	9	2^{9}	512
53	10	2^{10}	1024

Source: Model based on Sapareto and Dewey.[13]

From Table 4.1, one minute of heating at 48°C provides the same percentage cell kill as 32 minutes of heating at 43°C. One minute of heating at 49°C is equivalent to 64 minutes of heating at 43°C. To obtain an accurate thermal dose for the entire treatment region, multiple thermal sensors ideally should measure the thermal dose over the treatment volume, but in practice a single temperature sensor centrally placed in treatment volume might be sufficient to achieve the desired tumor cell kill.

As discussed in Chapter 2, Section 2.2, for 100% carcinoma cell kill for in vitro cells, it might be necessary to heat the cells, for example, at 48°C for a *minimum* of about 8 to 9 minutes. From Table 4.1, the equivalent minutes thermal dose (relative to 43°C heating) for this temperature (48°C) and duration of heating (8 to 9 minutes) has a range of $8 \times 32 = 256$ equivalent minutes to $9 \times 32 = 288$ equivalent minutes.

4.6 DETAILED MICROWAVE SPECIFIC ABSORPTION RATE CALCULATIONS IN SIMULATED BREAST TISSUE AND SIMULATED BREAST TUMORS

To estimate the heating pattern in normal breast tissue, and in normal breast tissue with tumor tissue exposed to focused microwave radiation, three-dimensional SAR heating patterns were calculated based on finite-difference time-domain (FDTD) theory and computer simulations developed by Taflove[15] at Northwestern University. In applying the FDTD method to thermotherapy treatments, the microwave applicators, tissues, and surrounding air are modeled by small cubes, and the electromagnetic field amplitude and phase at each cube is computed as a function of time based on Maxwell's electromagnetic field equations until steady-state fields are achieved. Referring to Equation 2.3, once the steady-state electromagnetic field distribution has been computed, the SAR distribution is then calculated from the magnitude of the E-field squared multiplied by the ionic conductivity of each cube—variation in tissue density is ignored in this model.

As depicted in **Figure 4.8**, dual-opposing waveguide applicators (TEM-2 applicators, Celsion (Canada) Limited, Ontario, Canada) operating at 915 MHz were modeled using the FDTD method. The applicators were coherently combined (common oscillator and phase tuned) to focus the radiated beam at the central position in 6-cm-thick homogeneous normal breast tissue (mixture of fat and glandular tissue with dielectric constant 12.5 and ionic conductivity 0.21 S/m). The applicators are assumed to radiate through thin sheets of rigid acrylic material that simulate the plates used for breast compression in the adaptive phased array breast thermotherapy system.

The side walls of each TEM-2 metallic waveguide are loaded with high dielectric constant material, which is used to match and shape the radiation inside the waveguide aperture. The waveguide applicators are linearly polarized with the alignment of the E-field in the y direction as in Figure 4.8. As shown in Figures 1.5 and 4.8, in a typical focused microwave thermotherapy treatment, the E-field polarization is aligned with the direction from the nipple to the base (chest wall) of the breast. For this geometry, the focused microwave energy propagates in a direction approximately parallel to the chest wall. Little microwave energy would be expected to penetrate the chest wall because the microwave reflection coefficient at low incidence angles is very high. The metallic waveguide walls are modeled with a dielectric constant 1.0 and ionic conductivity 3.7×10^7 S/m. In the FDTD computer simulation, a 5-mm flat sheet of acrylic material (dielectric constant 2.6, ionic conductivity 0.00013 S/m) is adjacent to each applicator and parallel to the waveguide aperture. Between the two opposing TEM-2 applicators is a 6-cm-thick homogeneous normal breast tissue phantom. The remaining volume is filled with 0.5-cm $\times$ 0.5-cm $\times$ 0.5-cm cubic cells that model air (dielectric constant 1.0, ionic conductivity 0.0 S/m).

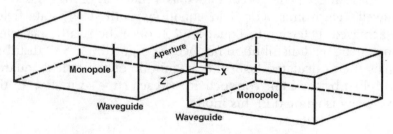

Figure 4.8 Geometry showing dual-opposing microwave waveguide applicators.

The SAR distributions in the simulated compressed breast were calculated by squaring the electric field amplitude and multiplying by the electrical conductivity of the simulated tissue (refer to Equation 2.3). SAR is often described in levels (50% is usually designated as the effective heating zone) relative to the maximum SAR value of 100%. The SAR is proportional to the initial rise in temperature per unit time, ignoring blood flow and thermal conduction effects.

The SAR patterns were computed in the three principal planes (xy, xz, yz) as shown in **Figures 4.9 to 4.11** for homogeneous normal breast tissue. The calculated SAR side (lateral) view (xy plane, $z = 0$) pattern (75% and 50% SAR contours) in homogeneous normal breast tissue is shown in Figure 4.9. The Figure 4.9 SAR pattern generally is bell shaped and centered between the TEM-2 applicators. Figure 4.10 shows the top view (xz plane, $y = 0$) SAR pattern (75% and 50% SAR contours). The Figure 4.10 SAR pattern exhibits a small elliptically shaped 75% SAR region surrounded by an elongated 50% SAR region. Figure 4.11 shows the end (cranial-caudal) view (yz plane, $x = 0$) of the SAR pattern (75% and 50% contours). The pattern exhibits a small circularly shaped 75% SAR region surrounded by an elongated 50% SAR region approximately the size of the waveguide aperture.

The results shown in Figures 4.9 to 4.11 indicate that a large volume of deep breast tissues can be heated by the adaptive phased array with focused TEM-2 waveguide applicators, whereas the superficial tissues are not substantially heated. Any high-water-content tissues exposed to this large heating field will be preferentially heated compared to the surrounding normal breast tissue as demonstrated in the following paragraphs.

To demonstrate selective (preferential) heating, two spherically shaped 1.5-cm-diameter simulated tumors (dielectric constant 58.6, electrical conductivity 1.05 S/m for breast carcinoma as listed in Table 2.1) were embedded in the normal phantom breast tissue with 5-cm spacing, and the FDTD SAR calculation for the top view is shown in **Figure 4.12**. From a comparison of this result with Figure 4.10, it is clear that the SAR contour pattern has changed significantly and the two high-water-content tumor regions are selectively heated. To quantitatively show the sharpness of the selective heating, the calculated SAR pattern cut along the z axis at $x = 0$ cm is shown in **Figure 4.13**. There is a sharp peak located at the position of each of the two

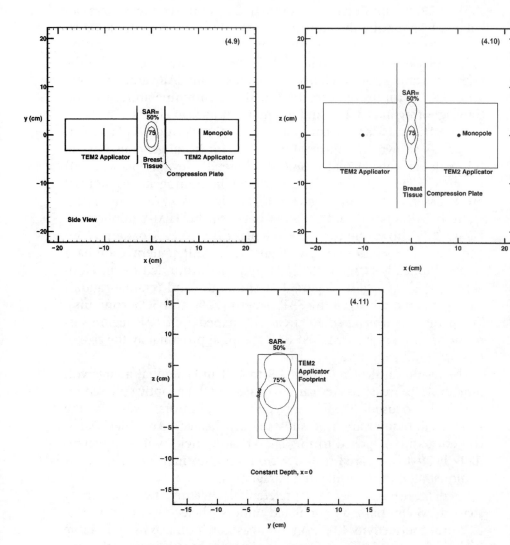

Figure 4.9   Calculated SAR contour pattern in the xy plane, $z = 0$, using the finite-difference time-domain method for dual-opposing TEM-2 waveguide applicators focused at the central position in simulated homogeneous normal breast tissue.

Figure 4.10   Calculated SAR contour pattern in the xz plane, $y = 0$, using the finite-difference time-domain method for dual-opposing TEM-2 waveguide applicators focused at the central position in simulated homogeneous normal breast tissue.

Figure 4.11   Calculated SAR contour pattern in the yz plane, $x = 0$, using the finite-difference time-domain method for dual-opposing TEM-2 waveguide applicators focused at the central position in simulated homogeneous normal breast tissue.

tumors, again demonstrating selective heating of the simulated high-water-, high-ion-content breast carcinoma compared to the surrounding normal breast tissue. Finally, a comparison of the SAR pattern cut along the x axis at $z = 0$ cm with and without tumor is shown in **Figure 4.14** — this cut traverses the central tumor at $z = 0$ and selective heating of the high-water-, high-ion-content tumor region is evident, when compared to the SAR pattern with no tumor present. Similar selective heating results would be expected for benign breast lesions such as fibroadenomas and cysts because they tend to have high water and high ion content, similar to breast carcinomas.

4.7 ADAPTIVE PHASED ARRAY ALGORITHM FOR FOCUSED MICROWAVE THERMOTHERAPY

A general-purpose multichannel adaptive phased array algorithm based on a gradient search technique for controlling microwave power and phase during thermotherapy treatments has been developed.[4-6] An adaptive phased array algorithm for rapidly adjusting the relative phase between two channels is described in this section.

As shown earlier in Figure 3.1, in a two-channel focused microwave thermotherapy system, only one phase shifter requires a relative phase adjustment, with respect to the other phase shifter, to achieve a microwave-focused condition. As shown in Figure 4.6, as the relative microwave phase ϕ changes over 360 degrees, the specific absorption rate in the tumor varies from a minimum to a maximum, with the minimum corresponding to a completely unfocused condition and the maximum SAR corresponding to a focused condition. As shown in Equation 4.9, the specific absorption rate is proportional to the electric-field squared or, equivalently, the microwave power measured by an electric-field probe positioned within a tumor. Let the measured microwave power received by the microwave probe be denoted as p^{rec}. A brute-force focusing approach would be to adjust the relative microwave phase in small phase increments (for example, 1 degree) over the full 360 degrees, and then measure the received microwave power p^{rec} at each phase increment. For example, for an arbitrary breast tissue thickness and arbitrary tumor depth, if the phase increment (denoted $\Delta\phi$) is 1 degree, it would take 360 phase adjustments and 360 power measurements to decide when the SAR maximum occurs. When the measured

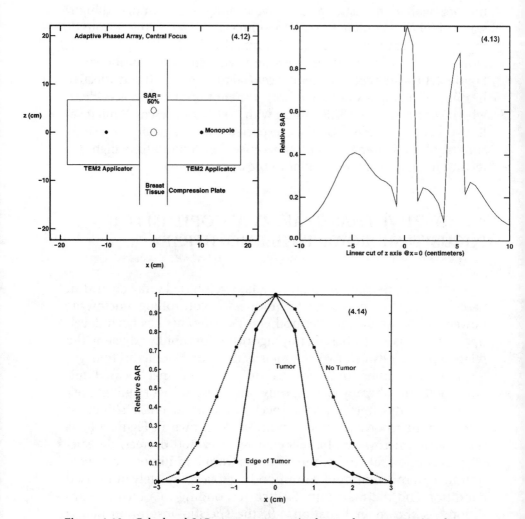

Figure 4.12   Calculated SAR contour pattern in the *xz* plane, *y* = 0, using the finite-difference time-domain method for dual-opposing TEM-2 waveguide applicators focused at the central position in simulated homogeneous normal breast tissue with two embedded spherically shaped 1.5-cm diameter simulated breast tumors.

Figure 4.13   Calculated SAR contour pattern cut along the *z* axis, *x* = 0 cm, using the finite-difference time-domain method for dual-opposing TEM-2 waveguide applicators focused at the central position in simulated homogeneous normal breast tissue (6 cm thick) with two embedded spherically shaped 1.5-cm diameter simulated breast tumors.

Figure 4.14   Calculated SAR contour pattern cut along the *x* axis, *z* = 0 cm, using the finite-difference time-domain method for dual-opposing TEM-2 waveguide applicators focused at the central position in simulated homogeneous normal breast tissue (6 cm thick) with and without two embedded spherically shaped 1.5-cm diameter simulated breast tumors.

microwave power p^{rec} is a maximum, the corresponding phase at which the maximum occurs is the desired phase-focusing condition. Such a brute-force focusing approach can be slow because of the time required to adjust the phase and then measure the corresponding received microwave power.

A faster approach is a method of steepest ascent gradient search algorithm that automatically searches for the correct phase setting that maximizes the received microwave power, and then the algorithm stops. Because of electromagnetic interference and noise, the measurement of microwave power by the probe in the tumor for small phase increments can have random fluctuations that could cause the algorithm to converge slowly and take at least 50 to 100 iterations to converge.

To reduce random fluctuations, it is possible to perform a series of microwave power measurements and average the data to improve the accuracy of the power measurement with a corresponding longer time to perform the phase-focusing operation and a reduction in the number of required iterations. Another method to speed the convergence of the gradient search is to include a fast acceleration term, which can reduce the number of iterations to just a few (less than about 5 primary iterations). A fast acceleration gradient search works as follows.[16]

Let there be a series of primary iterations (microwave phase settings) with index ranging from 1 to J, where the index at the jth primary iteration is denoted as j. Furthermore, for each primary iteration, let there be a subiteration index denoted k. At the jth iteration, the relative change (gradient) in received microwave power $\Delta p^{rec}{}_j$ is computed, in terms of a finite difference, as the phase shifter setting ϕ is dithered up and down in phase $(\pm \Delta \phi)$ and the absolute power is measured for each case, or

$$\Delta p^{rec}{}_j = p^{rec}{}_j (\phi_j + \Delta \phi) - p^{rec}{}_j (\phi_j - \Delta \phi) \qquad (4.19)$$

If $p^{rec}{}_j > 0$, then to maximize the received microwave power, the microwave phase should be adjusted in the positive phase direction. If $p^{rec}{}_j < 0$, then to maximize the received microwave power the microwave phase should be adjusted in the negative phase direction. Thus, the required gradient search direction, denoted r, can be computed as

$$r = \Delta p^{rec}{}_j \div \left| \Delta p^{rec}{}_j \right| \qquad (4.20)$$

where $|\ |$ represents absolute value.

Based on Equation 4.20, r takes on the value of either plus one $(+1)$ or minus one (-1) to indicate the desired search direction for the microwave phase to focus the array. Thus, for the adaptive phased array algorithm during the jth iteration of the phase adjustment, once the desired search direction (± 1 in this instance) is determined, the new phase increment during the subiterations ($k = 1, 2, 3, ...$) can take on the series of values $\Delta\phi$, $2\Delta\phi$, $4\Delta\phi$, ... , $2^{k-1}\Delta\phi$. During these subiterations, the phase is commanded to take on the values.

$$\phi_{j,k} = \phi_j + r\,2^{k-1}\Delta\phi, \; k = 1, 2, 3 \,... \tag{4.21}$$

and during these subiterations while the new phase is set the microwave power received at the microwave probe in the tumor is measured and compared to the previous value. If $p^{rec}_{j,k+1} > p^{rec}_{j,k}$, then the microwave received power is increasing and the focus is improving, so the subiteration procedure continues. If $p^{rec}_{j,k+1} < p^{rec}_{j,k}$, then the microwave received power is decreasing and the focus is not improving, so the subiteration procedure stops and the main iteration index j is then incremented to $j + 1$ and the algorithm continues resuming with Equations 4.19 to 4.21 until the maximum value of received microwave power is determined. A typical value for the phase increment $\Delta\phi$ can be, say, 5 degrees throughout the entire focusing algorithm, or this value can be changed (decreased) depending on the overall system design, taking account of the quantization and random errors in measuring the received microwave power as well as in setting the desired phase shifter values.

4.8 SUMMARY

This chapter has reviewed the physics for understanding and quantifying the transcutaneous delivery of focused microwave phased array energy to the breast. Background on the generation of microwaves and the addition of microwaves from multiple coherent antenna radiators (a phased array) was reviewed. A simplified theory and analysis for focused microwave energy propagating through breast tissue were presented. The computation of both microwave energy dose and tissue thermal dose was reviewed. A detailed three-dimensional finite-difference time-domain electromagnetic analysis of a focused microwave phased array applicator system for treatment of breast cancer demonstrated selective heating of tumors in simulated breast tissues. An adaptive phased array focusing algorithm for real-time control during focused microwave thermotherapy has been reviewed. The next chapter describes preclinical results for focused microwave thermotherapy.

REFERENCES

1. Kraus JD. *Electromagnetics*. New York, NY: McGraw-Hill; 1953:347–518.
2. Lee ER. Electromagnetic superficial heating technology. In: Seegenschmiedt MH, Fessenden P, Vernon CC, eds. *Thermo-Radiotherapy and Thermo-Chemotherapy*. New York, NY: Springer-Verlag; 1995;1:119–217.
3. von Hippel AR, Runck AH, Westphal WB. *Dielectric Analysis of Biomaterials*. Cambridge, Mass: Massachusetts Institute of Technology, Laboratory for Insulation Research; 1973:16–20. Technical Report 13, AD-769 843.
4. Fenn AJ. Adaptive nulling hyperthermia array. US Patent Number 5,251,645. October 12, 1993.
5. Fenn AJ, King GA. Experimental investigation of an adaptive feedback algorithm for hot spot reduction in radio-frequency phased-array hyperthermia. *IEEE Trans Biomed Eng.* 1994;43(3):273–280.
6. Fenn AJ, Wolf GL, Fogle RM. An adaptive phased array for targeted heating of deep tumors in intact breast: animal study results. *Int J Hyperthermia.* 1999;15(1):45–61.
7. Gauthrie M, ed. *Methods of External Hyperthermic Heating*. New York, NY: Springer-Verlag; 1990:8.
8. Field SB, Hand JW. *An Introduction to the Practical Aspects of Clinical Hyperthermia*. New York, NY: Taylor & Francis; 1990:290.
9. Fenn AJ, Bornstein BA, Svensson GK, Bowman HF. Minimally invasive monopole phased arrays for hyperthermia treatment of breast carcinomas: design and phantom tests. *Int Symp on Electromagnetic Compatibility* (Sendai, Japan). 1994;(10)2:566–569.
10. Chaudhary SS, Mishra RK, Swarup A, Thomas JM. Dielectric properties of normal and malignant human breast tissue at radiowave and microwave frequencies. *Indian J Biochem Biophys.* 1984;21:76–79.
11. Joines WT, Zhang Y, Li C, Jirtle RL. The measured electrical properties of normal and malignant human tissues from 50 to 900 MHz. *Med Phys.* 1994;21(4):547–550.

12. Vitrogan D. *Elements of Electric and Magnetic Circuits*. San Francisco, Calif: Rinehart Press; 1971:31–34.

13. Sapareto SA, Dewey WC. Thermal dose determination in cancer therapy. *Int J Rad Oncol Biol Phys*. 1984;10:787–800.

14. Jones EL, Oleson JR, Prosnitz LR, et al. Randomized trial of hyperthermia and radiation for superficial tumors. *J Clin Oncol*. 2005;23(13):3079–3085.

15. Taflove A. *Computational Electrodynamics: The Finite-Difference Time-Domain Method*. Norwood, Mass: Artech House; 1995.

16. Fenn AJ. Thermodynamic adaptive phased array system for activating thermosensitive liposomes in targeted drug delivery. US Patent Number 5,810,888. September 22, 1998.

PROBLEM SET

4.1 Using Equations 4.5 and 4.8, use computer software to calculate the microwave attenuation at 915 MHz for each of the tissues listed in Table 2.1.

4.2 Using Equations 4.5 and 4.6, at 915 MHz for homogeneous normal breast tissue (with approximate dielectric constant 12.5 and electrical conductivity 0.21 S/m), verify that the calculated attenuation constant α is 0.11 radians/cm and the phase propagation constant β is 0.69 radians/cm, or 39.5 electrical degrees per cm. Then, using Equation 4.7, verify that the wavelength in homogeneous normal breast tissue is approximately 9.0 cm at 915 MHz, and from Equation 4.8 verify that the microwave loss is approximately 1 dB/cm.

4.3 Use Equations 4.1a and 4.1b and computer software to verify the results in Figure 4.5 that depict unfocused and focused microwave examples in which two 915 MHz microwaves with unity amplitude incident at the focal point $(x = 0)$ are either constantly out of phase by a relative phase shift of $\phi(t) = 135°$ or they are constantly in phase $\phi(t) = 0°$.

4.4. Verify that Equation 4.11 follows from Equations 4.9 and 4.10.

4.5. Verify that Equations 4.13 and 4.15 follow from Equations 4.12 and 4.14, respectively.

4.6 Assuming 6-cm breast tissue thickness and dual opposing 915-MHz microwave applicators, use computer software to program Equations 4.13 and 4.15 and compute the SAR on the left and right skin surfaces and in the central tissue site (tumor) as the relative phase shift of Channel 2 (ϕ_2) varies from -180 degrees to $+180$ degrees and verify the results shown in Figure 4.6.

4.7 Equation 4.18 (equivalent minutes thermal dose relative to 43°C) is easily programmed in one line using Microsoft Excel. For example, the code

```
=SUM(IF((A1:A10)<43,0.25,0.5)^(43-A1:A10))*0.5
```

calculates the cumulative equivalent minutes thermal dose for a given column (A1:A10) of temperature measurements taken one-half minute (0.5 minutes) apart. Verify with Microsoft Excel, or other computer software such as MATLAB (The MathWorks, Inc.), that the simple case of a constant temperature of 44 degrees Celsius for five (5) minutes yields an equivalent thermal dose of ten (10) minutes.

Preclinical Results for Focused Microwave Phased Array Thermotherapy for Treating the Intact Breast

5.1 INTRODUCTION

Prior to conducting human clinical studies, it was necessary to perform tests to demonstrate the safety and performance of the adaptive phased array thermotherapy system for treating the intact compressed breast. As an approximate model for an intact female breast, thermotherapy tests were conducted on a nonperfused breast phantom (Section 5.2), small animals (rabbits) (Section 5.3), and larger animals (pigs) (Section 5.4) that included blood perfusion effects. Compression of the treated tissue was not used in the rabbit study, whereas the pig study included the effects of breast compression plates.A two-channel microwave thermotherapy system with adaptive phase control (Microfocus-1000 APA System, Celsion [Canada] Limited, Ontario, Canada) was used in the preclinical studies—a block diagram of the adaptive phased array thermotherapy system is shown in Figure 3.2. Each channel provided up to 100 watts of microwave power at 915 MHz (megahertz). The amplifiers were driven from a common oscillator, and electronically controlled phase shifters enabled the relative phase difference between the two channels to be varied. Two linearly polarized, dielectric-slab-loaded, rectangular waveguide applicators[1] (Model TEM-2, Celsion [Canada] Limited) were used to induce thermotherapy. The overall dimensions of the aperture of these TEM-2 applicators were 6.5 cm (parallel to the electric field) by 13 cm (perpendicular to the electric field). The aperture of the air-filled region between the dielectric slabs was 6.5 cm × 9.0 cm. Air cooling of the skin was provided through the air-filled region of the applicator aperture by means of a fan mounted behind a perforated electrically conducting screen at the back of the applicator.

5.2 BREAST PHANTOM TESTING

To demonstrate selective tumor heating with a focused microwave phased array breast thermotherapy system, a simulated breast tumor mass of variable size was embedded in simulated normal breast tissue and the specific absorption rate (SAR) pattern was measured. **Figure 5.1** shows a side view of the externally focused adaptive phased array thermotherapy applicators with breast compression plates (3-cm-thick acrylic) on either side of a multislice breast phantom that is used to simulate the breast for microwave heating SAR experiments.

The breast phantom contained fatty dough material (approximately 66.7% flour, 30.0% oil, and 3.3% NaCl solution [0.9% NaCl per liter of water] by weight) described by Lagendijk[2] with microwave properties similar to normal breast tissue. The breast tumor was simulated with high-water-content muscle phantom tissue (approximately 75.2% water, 1.0% NaCl, 15.4% Polyethylene powder, and 8.4% TX-151 gelling agent) described by Chou et al.[3] The 6-cm-thick breast phantom was constructed out of six slices using acrylic frames — each frame provided a 1-cm-thick slice simulating normal breast tissue with a simulated 2-cm-thick cancerous breast tumor modeled in the two central frames. The slices were numbered 1 through 6, with slices 1 and 6 being the surface slices, and slices 3 and 4 the central slices.

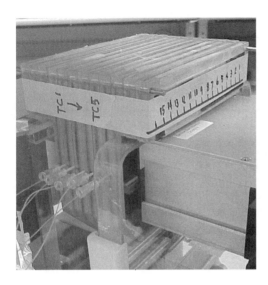

Figure 5.1 Photograph showing a multi-slice breast phantom, compression plates, and dual opposing microwave applicators.

Photo courtesy of Celsion (Canada) Limited.

Five thermocouple (TC) catheter tracts spaced 1 cm apart (located between the slices) and labeled TC1, TC2, TC3, TC4, and TC5 were used and had subsurface depths of 1 cm, 2 cm, 3 cm, 2 cm, and 1 cm, respectively. TC probes (Physitemp Instruments, Inc, Clifton, New Jersey) were inserted in the catheters and were moved linearly using a computer-controlled probe scanning mechanism to 15 positions that were 1 cm apart.

A drawing of central phantom slice number 3 is shown in **Figure 5.2** with an example tumor modeled, having width L_z, at the approximate center of the slice. An E-field sensor probe (coaxial cable with the center pin extended) was placed with the tip at the approximate central depth of the tumor. A catheter for the TC sensor was placed laterally in the tumor and was perpendicular to the E-field polarization. In Figure 5.2, the E-field probe catheter tract is denoted by the letter E, and the TC sensor catheter tract is denoted by the letter T. In each of three different experiments, the two middle sections (slices 3 and 4) contained equal-size tumor phantom ($1 \text{ cm} \times 2 \text{ cm} \times 2$ cm, $1 \text{ cm} \times 2 \text{ cm} \times 6$ cm, or $1 \text{ cm} \times 2 \text{ cm} \times 8$ cm) so that when the two slices were placed together, central tumor masses with approximate elliptical dimensions ($L_x = 2$, $L_y = 2$, $L_z = 2$ cm), ($L_x = 2$, $L_y = 2$, $L_z = 6$ cm), or ($L_x = 2$, $L_y = 2$, $L_z = 8$ cm) were modeled (refer to Figure 4.8 for the x, y, z axis orientations).

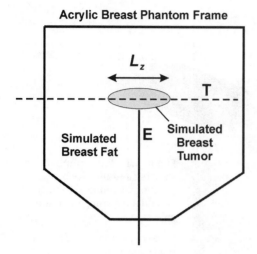

Acrylic Breast Phantom Frame

L_z

T

E

Simulated
Breast Fat

Simulated
Breast
Tumor

Figure 5.2 Drawing of a central breast phantom slice, 1 cm thick, with an E-field sensor catheter and temperature sensor catheter inserted in an example simulated breast tumor.

Heating was performed at 50 watts per channel over 20-second bursts with 20 minutes between measurements to allow the phantom temperature to return to equilibrium—a complete set of measurements for the 15 probe positions in the catheters took approximately 5 hours. The SAR was calculated by the rise in temperature at each measurement position over the 20-second heating interval, and then was plotted as normalized SAR with a peak value of 1.0. A normalized SAR value of 0.5 (50%) is typically used to estimate the effective heating zone.

The microwave applicators are designed for clinical treatments so that a gap region (typically 1 cm or more) is provided between the applicator and the breast tissue. The gap region allows air to flow from external air tubes or fans that are pointed into the gap to cool the region in proximity to the skin and base of each side of the breast and chest wall region. For phantom testing, air cooling was not used.

The adaptive microwave phased array thermotherapy system was focused using the E-field probe sensor in the simulated tumor as the feedback signal. The measured SAR profile results for the three different tumor sizes (2 cm, 6 cm, and 8 cm width) are shown in **Figure 5.3**. The SAR heating zone selectively expands in size according to the tumor size and encompasses nearly the entire tumor mass. Therefore, the measured data show that the desired selective heating of a high-water-content simulated homogeneous tumor mass is

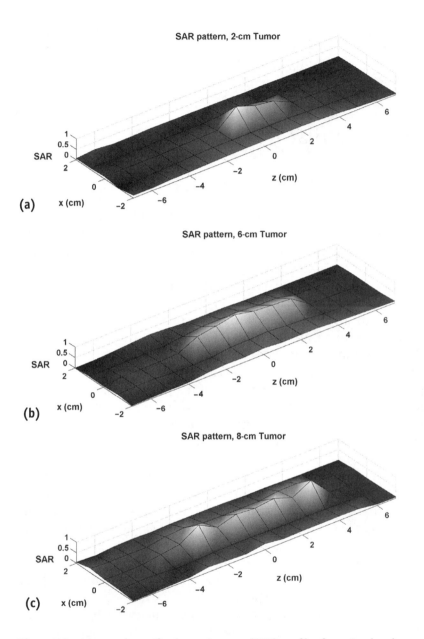

Figure 5.3 Measured specific absorption rate (SAR) profiles for a simulated compressed breast phantom with breast carcinoma of variable size. The width of the effective heating zone is approximately equal to the width of the simulated tumor. (a) $2 \times 2 \times 2$ cm simulated breast tumor. (b) $2 \times 2 \times 6$ cm simulated breast tumor. (c) $2 \times 2 \times 8$ cm simulated breast tumor.

achieved in a nonperfused breast phantom. Based on these measured phantom data, the focused microwave phased array thermotherapy system is capable of heating breast tumors that can vary in size from small to large diameter.

5.3 SMALL ANIMAL TESTING

5.3.1 Methods and Materials

Thermotherapy testing of the adaptive phased array breast thermotherapy system was conducted in small animals from March 1997 to May 1998 at the Massachusetts General Hospital Center for Imaging and Pharmaceutical Research.[4] The in vivo trials were conducted in several New Zealand White rabbits. The study was approved by the Subcommittee on Research Animal Care and conducted in an Association for Assessment and Accreditation of Laboratory Animal Care–accredited facility.

The rabbit hind leg provides a model of perfused muscle tissue in the thigh region with a subcutaneous fat layer in the range of 2 to 3 mm thick. As mentioned in Chapter 2, Section 2 (Table 2.1), muscle is significantly more difficult to penetrate with microwaves (915-MHz microwave loss = 2.9 dB/cm) compared to normal breast tissue (915-MHz microwave loss = 1 dB/cm). Thus, for demonstrating breast tumor heating in 4- to 8-cm-thick compressed breast tissue, these tests in microwave-lossy muscle tissue can represent more difficult heating conditions compared to human trials. The animals were anesthetized with halothane prior to setup of the experiments and clinically monitored during the treatments. Experiments with single microwave thermotherapy applicators and adaptive microwave phased array thermotherapy applicators opposing the hind leg were conducted in animals with and without tumors. All animals were euthanized via lethal injection following the treatments.

Figure 5.4 shows the animal trial test geometry for heating comparisons between the dual-opposing adaptive phased array microwave applicators and the single microwave applicator. Note: Breast compression plates were not used in these experiments because compression of the rabbit hind leg was not required.

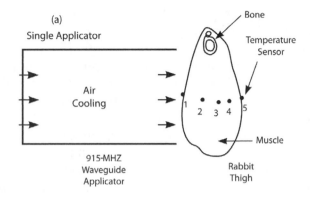

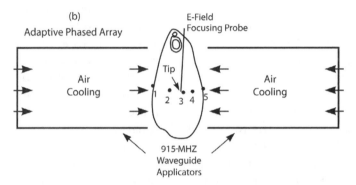

Figure 5.4 Thermotherapy animal trials experimental configurations for heating rabbit hind leg. **(a)** Single applicator, and **(b)** adaptive phased array applicators for focused microwave thermotherapy.

Source: Fenn AJ, Wolf GL, and Fogle RM. An adaptive microwave phased array for targeted heating of deep tumors in intact breast: animal study results. *Int J Hyperthermia* 1999;15(1):45–61. www.tandf.co.uk/journals. Used with permission from Taylor & Francis.

The animal trials used up to five TC temperature probes (Physitemp Instruments, Inc., Clifton, New Jersey)—these probes are denoted 1, 2, 3, 4, 5. In each experiment, the rabbit hind leg thickness was approximately 4 cm and the spacing between the temperature probes was approximately 1 cm. Temperature probes 1 and 5 were positioned on the opposing skin surfaces of the hind leg. The hind leg was shaved, so that the skin-surface-mounted TC probes could be taped to the skin and accurately contact and measure the temperatures of the skin. The E-field probe and temperature probes 2, 3, 4 were inserted into the tissue within closed-end plastic catheters. Probes 2 and 4 were at a depth of about 1 cm and probe 3 was at the focal depth of 2 cm. The tips of all probes were approximately aligned with the projected midpoint of the waveguide apertures. The temperature probes were aligned approximately perpendicular to the electric-field polarization of the 915-MHz waveguide applicators so that they would not scatter significant amounts of microwave energy during treatments or not be significantly heated by the microwave field. To focus the dual-applicator phased array thermotherapy system adaptively, the E-field probe was inserted into the central tissue position (2-cm depth) approximately parallel to and strongly coupled with the electric field radiated by the applicators.

For the dual opposing adaptively focused microwave phased array, the 915-MHz electronic phase shifters were adjusted typically in a total of 5 to 10 seconds using an adaptive phased array algorithm[5] with acceleration to focus the microwave radiation rapidly at the central tissue site. The locations of all probes were verified using an X-ray computerized tomography scan prior to each treatment. Note: In clinical practice, as described in Chapters 6 through 9, the orientation of the E-field probe and temperature probe in the breast is verified using ultrasound imaging. The two 915-MHz microwave applicators used air cooling (room temperature air, 20°C) to limit the amount of heating induced in the skin. For these tests, the target feedback temperature of centrally located temperature probe 3 was 43°C for 60-minute treatments or 46°C for shorter-duration treatments.

5.3.2 Results

A few initial experimental safety tests allowed limited comparisons to be made between a conventional single microwave TEM-2 applicator (Figure 5.4[a]) and the adaptive phased array method with dual microwave TEM-2 applicators (Figure 5.4[b]) for heating the animal hind leg. For comparison purposes, the procedure required that the same leg and the same temperature probe positions be used. Experiments in the animals were performed in the following manner. First, the hind leg was heated for a 60-minute treatment session with the phase shifters of the dual-applicator adaptive phased array adjusted to focus on and heat the central tissue position (2-cm deep).

Then, the microwave generator was turned off and the leg was allowed to cool (for approximately 45 minutes) back to normal body temperature. During the period when the microwave equipment was turned off, one of the applicators was removed as depicted in Figure 5.4(a). Finally, without disturbing the initial test configuration, the microwave system was turned back on and a single applicator under automatic power control heated the same leg for 60 minutes. The same microwave power control algorithm was used to control the power delivered to either the adaptive phased array or the single applicator.

For the higher-temperature tests, the adaptive phased array thermotherapy configuration was the same as shown in Figure 5.4(b) except that only three temperature probes (probes 1, 3, and 5) were used, that is, one probe was in the tumor (probe 3) and two probes were on the skin surface (probes 1 and 5). The feedback temperature was set to achieve and maintain 46°C in the tumor for 8 minutes.

The contrast between a focused microwave phased array thermotherapy treatment and a single-applicator treatment is shown in **Figures 5.5** and **5.6**. Figure 5.5 (adaptive phased array treatment) and Figure 5.6 (single-applicator treatment) show the measured temperatures versus time and commanded applicator power versus time. For the dual-applicator adaptive phased array, it is observed in Figure 5.5 that the target feedback temperature (probe 3) is achieved in only about 4 minutes, that after a minor oscillatory behavior at 43°C (±0.5°C) lasting about 16 minutes the temperature stabilizes at 43°C (±0.1°C) for a 40-minute period, and that the calculated equivalent thermal dose was 49.5 minutes relative to 43°C. During the stabilized heating period, probe 2 temperature is about 44°C and probe 4 temperature is about 41°C. It should be observed that the skin temperatures are maintained below about 33°C. The adaptive phased array microwave power level, to maintain 43°C at the feedback probe, is only about 3 watts (W).

For the single applicator, in Figure 5.6 the desired 43°C feedback temperature (probe 3) is achieved in about 10 minutes; however, excessive heating at the probe 2 position (1 cm beneath the skin surface adjacent to the radiating applicator) above 50°C is observed. In addition, the single microwave applicator-induced skin temperatures are elevated to the range of between 33° and 39°C. The microwave power level is oscillatory and has a maximum above 50 W. In this

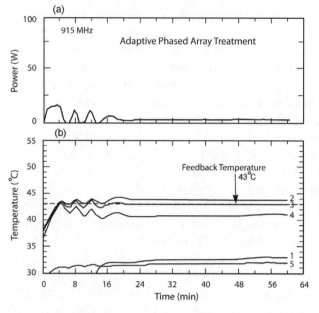

Figure 5.5

(a) microwave power and **(b)** temperature for dual-applicator adaptive microwave phased array heating rabbit hind leg. The feedback temperature is 43°C.

Source: Fenn AJ, Wolf GL, and Fogle RM. An adaptive microwave phased array for targeted heating of deep tumors in intact breast: animal study results. *Int J Hyperthermia* 1999;15(1):45–61. www.tandf.co.uk/journals. Used with permission from Taylor & Francis.

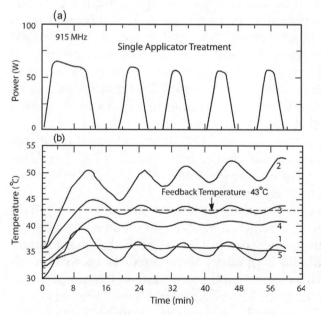

Figure 5.6

(a) microwave power and **(b)** temperature for single applicator heating rabbit hind leg. The feedback temperature is 43°C.

Source: Fenn AJ, Wolf GL, and Fogle RM. An adaptive microwave phased array for targeted heating of deep tumors in intact breast: animal study results. *Int J Hyperthermia* 1999;15(1):45–61. www.tandf.co.uk/journals. Used with permission from Taylor & Francis.

experiment, uncontrolled excessive heating at probe 2 is likely caused by the absorption of a substantial amount of microwave energy as the microwave signal propagates through the superficial tissue.

An experiment with the adaptive phased array using the target feedback temperature of 46°C at the tumor for 8 minutes was conducted. **Figure 5.7** shows the microwave power and temperature versus time data and demonstrates that the desired feedback temperature is achieved after approximately 8 minutes of heating and is then maintained for the desired 8-minute time interval. The tumor equivalent thermal dose delivered was 91.7 minutes relative to 43°C. During the entire treatment interval, the skin temperatures were below 35°C and the average microwave power per applicator was in the range of 25 to 30 W.

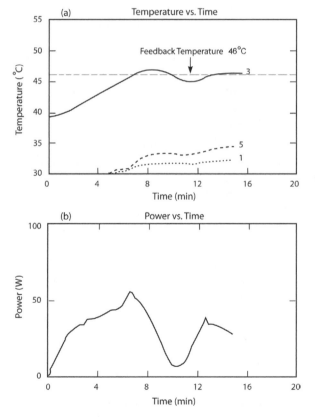

Figure 5.7

Dual-opposing applicator adaptive microwave phased array heating rabbit hind leg. The feedback temperature is 46°C.

(a) Measured temperature in tumor and at superficial sites. (b) Commanded microwave power

Source: Fenn AJ, Wolf GL, and Fogle RM. An adaptive microwave phased array for targeted heating of deep tumors in intact breast: animal study results. *Int J Hyperthermia* 1999;15(1):45-61. www.tandf.co.uk/journals. Used with permission from Taylor & Francis.

5.3.3 Discussion and Summary

In these preclinical tests of a Microfocus-1000 dual-opposing air-cooled adaptive microwave phased array thermotherapy system, a feedback temperature of either 43°C or 46°C was readily achieved at a central tissue depth in a rabbit hind leg model without excessive superficial heating. In contrast, the single unfocused microwave applicator exhibited excessive superficial heating of the rabbit hind leg while attempting to heat the central tissue depth.

The adaptive phased array experiment described here used two coherent microwave channels, containing electronically adjustable phase shifters to focus the microwave energy at an E-field feedback probe. This adaptive phased array system has significant advantage over a nonadaptive phased array. A nonadaptive phased array with two channels could, in theory, produce a null, a maximum, or an intermediate value of E-field depending on whether the two radiated waves are 180 degrees out-of-phase, completely in-phase, or partly out-of-phase, respectively. Because the adaptive phased array automatically focuses the E-field in the presence of all tissue-scattering structures, this type of array should provide more reliable deep-focused heating compared to manually adjusted or pretreatment planning–controlled phased arrays.

The ability of a dual-applicator adaptive microwave phased array to heat semideep tissues has been confirmed in a small live animal model of the breast. The experiments were performed in high-water-content perfused muscle tissue that theoretically is more difficult to heat at depth compared to the same thickness of low-water-content fatty breast tissue. Based on the measured data from these experiments in a rabbit hind leg, the adaptive microwave phased array breast thermotherapy system demonstrates the necessary safety to warrant additional investigations in humans as described in Chapters 6, 7, 8, and 9. However, prior to the start of human trials, additional tests in larger animals were conducted as reviewed in the next section.

5.4 LARGE ANIMAL TESTING

In this section, additional pre-clinical safety assessment of the heating capabilities of the two-channel 915 MHz Microfocus APA 1000 hyperthermia system with adaptive phase control is briefly described based on a study by Gavrilov et al.[6] These additional animal experiments were performed in the hind legs of pigs, which are significantly thicker (50% or greater) than the rabbit hind legs used in the previous small animal study[4] reviewed in Section 5.3. In addition, the large animal study includes the use of dielectric plates to compress the tissue, whereas the previous rabbit study did not require or utilize compression plates. Section 5.4.1 describes the methods and materials used in the large animal study, Section 5.4.2 describes the results, and Section 5.4.3 summarizes the study.

5.4.1 Methods and Materials

Focused microwave thermotherapy tests in large animals (pigs) were conducted in March to April 1998 at Oxford University in Oxford, England, in collaboration with Hammersmith Hospital in London as decribed by Gavrilov et al[6]. The aim of the study was to carry out an additional preclinical safety assessment of the heating capabilities of a two-channel 915-MHz focused microwave thermotherapy system with adaptive phase control. These additional animal experiments were performed in the hind legs of pigs, which are significantly thicker (50% or greater) than the rabbit hind legs used in the rabbit preclinical tests described in Section 5.3. The large animal study included the use of plastic plates to compress the tissue, whereas the previous rabbit study did not require or use compression plates.

Female English Large White pigs, aged 7 to 8 months and weighing 50 to 70 kg, were used in these preclinical tests that were conducted under veterinarian care. Prior to microwave heating, the animals were anaesthetized using a halothane (2–3%), nitrous oxide (30%), oxygen mixture and were intubated. They were positioned supinely during thermotherapy sessions.

The site treated in each animal was the muscle region of the hind leg. The leg was supported in a near vertical position. The dimensions of the legs (variation and range of muscle thickness, bone thickness) were measured and the borders of a bone-free volume of tissue were estimated to determine an appropriate treatment volume.

A two-channel microwave thermotherapy system with adaptive phase control (Microfocus APA 1000 system, Celsion [Canada] Limited, Ontario, Canada) was used in this study. Each channel provided up to 100 W of power at 915 MHz. The amplifiers were driven from a common oscillator, and electronically controlled phase shifters enabled the relative phase difference between channels to be varied. As described in Section 5.1, two linearly polarized, dielectric-slab-loaded, rectangular waveguide applicators (Model TEM-2, Celsion Canada, Limited) were used to induce thermotherapy. The apertures of the applicators were separated from the skin surface by fixing 4-mm-thick acrylic plates with numerous holes to maintain air-cooling capability across the fronts of the applicators.

An E-field probe, consisting of a length of semirigid coaxial cable (0.9-mm outside diameter) with the outer conductor removed to expose 1 cm of the central conductor at the tip, was implanted into the central region of tissue to be heated using a 1.5-mm outside diameter metal trocar and polytetrafluoroethylene catheter. This probe was used to measure the local E-field at the "target" location and to provide a signal that enabled the adaptive phase control algorithm to set the phase difference between channels that resulted in maximum (focused) E-field at that location in approximately 5 seconds.

Temperature sensing was carried out with six probes using two single-junction TCs and one multisensor (4 junctions) TC in which the intersensor spacing was 1 cm (Physitemp Instruments, Inc, Clifton, New Jersey). All of the TCs were copper-constantan type, enclosed within a 0.6-mm outside diameter Teflon catheter. For purposes of measuring the temperature versus depth in this animal study, the TC sensors were all aligned along a line through the focus connecting the midpoint of each of the dual-opposing applicator apertures—the dashed line shown in **Figure 5.8** is aligned with the linear path in tissue of the TC sensors. The two single-junction TCs (referred to later as probes 1 and 2) were used to measure the subcutaneous temperature. Probe 1 was positioned beneath the applicator on the outer side of the leg, and probe 2 was positioned on the inner side of the leg, both at depth of 2 mm (Figure 5.8). The four-junction TC was placed in the muscle using a trocar, which was inserted through the whole thickness of the muscle block. The TCs were aligned approximately perpendicular to the direction of the linearly polarized electric field produced by the applicators. The centrally positioned temperature probe provided a feedback signal to control the microwave power delivered to the applicators to set the desired target temperature.

Having determined an appropriate region and identified the positions in which the applicators would be placed, TCs were implanted in

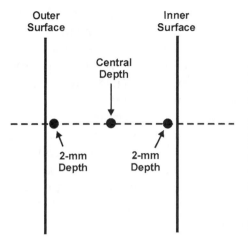

Figure 5.8 Location of temperature probes for pig hind leg heating tests.

Source: Adapted from Gavrilov LR, Hand JW, Hopewell JW, and Fenn AJ. Pre-clinical evaluation of a two-channel microwave hyperthermia system with adaptive phase control in a large animal, *Int J Hyperthermia* 1999;15(6):495–507. www.tandf.co.uk/journals. Used with permission from Taylor & Francis.

the manner described earlier. The muscle region within the treatment volume was then compressed using the two applicators positioned in a parallel-opposed arrangement similar to that shown in Figure 3.1. Typically, the microwave applicators were separated by a distance of 6.5 to 7 cm, although in larger animals the thickness of the compressed tissue region was greater and as much as 11 cm in one case.[6] The E-field focusing probe, aligned approximately parallel to the direction of polarization of the E-field, was implanted close to the central position of the muscle region. The central tissue target (feedback) temperature was set to 43°C for each experiment. Temperature measurements, phase shifting, and microwave power were monitored and controlled by a personal computer. The specific absorption rate at each of the temperature-monitored tissue sites was computed by the average rate of increase of temperature during the first 120 seconds of heating.

5.4.2 Results

Measured temperatures during treatment as a function of time, both at the center of the muscle (at 3.25 to 3.5 cm depth) and in the superficial surface tissues (outer surface probe 1 at 2 mm depth), in two animals (pig hind leg) with similar muscle thickness (6.5–7 cm) are shown in **Figure 5.9**. In these two cases, therapeutic temperatures approximately 43°C were achieved at central depth

while the temperatures recorded in more superficial tissues were 2°
to 3°C lower, particularly after 15 to 20 minutes from the beginning of the application of microwave power. To achieve the 43°C
central depth temperature the peak microwave power required was
approximately 40 W for each of the two animals.[6] The $CEM_{43°C}$
thermal equivalent thermal dose in minutes at 43°C at the central
tissue position (focus) and at the outer surface position of the hind
leg of pigs 1 and 2 was calculated using Equation 4.18. For both
pigs, a significant thermal dose (30.3 minutes, 25.9 minutes) was
delivered to the central tissue site, whereas very little thermal dose
(2.3 minutes, 0.9 minutes) was delivered to the outer surface position. Measurements were also performed for pigs #1 and #2 in
which the relative microwave phase between the two microwave applicators was intentionally offset from the ideal focused condition.[6]
For a 59-degree phase-focusing error, the ratio of the measured sub-

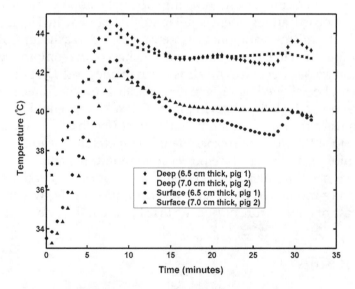

Figure 5.9   Measured temperature versus time at the center of the pig muscle
(3.25 to 3.5 cm deep) and in the superficial tissue (2 mm deep) for adaptively
focused microwave phased array experiments in two animals (pigs #1 and #2)
with similar muscle thickness (6.5–7 cm).

Source: Adapted from Gavrilov LR, Hand JW, Hopewell JW, and Fenn AJ. Pre-clinical evaluation of a two-channel microwave hyperthermia system with adaptive phase control in a large
animal, *Int J Hyperthermia* 1999;15(6):495–507. www.tandf.co.uk/journals. Used with permission from Taylor & Francis.

cutaneous (2 mm depth) SAR to central depth SAR increased by about 43%, and for a 127-degree phase-focusing error this ratio increased by about 80% compared to the ideal focused condition. From these measurements and also referring to the previous simulations in Figures 4.5 and 4.6, large phase focusing errors clearly would increase the likelihood of overheating superficial tissue and producing superficial burns that should be avoided during thermotherapy treatments.

5.4.3 Discussion and Summary

The results of the preclinical experiments using the Microfocus APA 1000 focused microwave thermotherapy system show that when the muscle region of the hind legs of pigs can be compressed to 6.5 to 7 cm, a pair of parallel opposed, coherently driven 915-MHz applicators can elevate the temperature in the central tissue to therapeutic levels without overheating superficial tissues when the phase difference between applicators is determined by the adaptive phase control algorithm. The results obtained support the potential of using the adaptive microwave phased array technique for thermotherapy treatment of centrally located breast tumors in a 4- to 8-cm-thick compressed breast, particularly because 915-MHz microwave attenuation is about 1 dB/cm for normal breast tissue and about 3 dB/cm (see Section 2.3.1) in muscle corresponding to the pig model. The results of this study demonstrate further safety for human clinical trials for breast cancer patients.

5.5 SUMMARY

This chapter has reviewed preclinical testing for understanding and quantifying the transcutaneous delivery of focused microwave energy to the breast. Animal tests in rabbit hind leg and pig hind leg demonstrated that adaptive phased array thermotherapy produced heating of semideep tissue while maintaining safe temperatures on the surface. The next four chapters describe clinical studies performed with focused microwave thermotherapy for female patients with breast cancer.

REFERENCES

1. Cheung AY, Dao T, Robinson JE. Dual-beam TEM applicator for direct-contact heating of dielectrically encapsulated malignant mouse tumor. *Radio Science.* 1977;12(6(S)suppl):81–85.

2. Lagendijk JJW, Nilsson P. Hyperthermia dough: a fat and bone equivalent phantom to test microwave/radiofrequency hyperthermia heating systems. *Phys Med Biol.* 1985;30(7):709–712.

3. Chou CK, Chen GW, Guy AW, Luk KH. Formulas for preparing phantom muscle tissue at various radiofrequencies. *Biolectromagnetics.* 1984;5:435–441.

4. Fenn AJ, Wolf GL, Fogle RM. An adaptive phased array for targeted heating of deep tumors in intact breast: animal study results. *Int J Hyperthermia.* 1999;15(1):45–61.

5. Fenn AJ, King GA. Experimental investigation of an adaptive feedback algorithm for hot spot reduction in radio-frequency phased-array hyperthermia. *IEEE Trans Biomed Eng.* 1994;43(3):273–280.

6. Gavrilov LR, Hand JW, Hopewell JW, Fenn AJ. Pre-clinical evaluation of a two-channel microwave hyperthermia system with adaptive phase control in a large animal. *Int J Hyperthermia.* 1999;15(6):495–507.

Clinical Results for Preoperative Focused Microwave Phased Array Thermotherapy Treatment of Cancer in the Intact Breast

PART

III

Phase I Safety Study of Focused Microwave Thermotherapy for Invasive Breast Carcinomas in Patients Scheduled for Mastectomy

6.1 INTRODUCTION

A small (10-patient) Phase I study by Gardner et al[1] was designed and conducted to establish the safety and feasibility of the use of preoperative focused microwave phased array thermotherapy for treating primary breast cancer. Patients treated under this Food and Drug Administration (FDA)–approved Phase I safety study were patients with breast cancer that were scheduled for mastectomy. The goal of this Phase I study was to determine whether a 60-minute equivalent thermal dose (relative to 43°C) could be used to safely heat, damage, and reduce the size of primary breast carcinomas prior to surgery. In this study, all patients received a mastectomy regardless of any tumor response to thermotherapy. It was expected that the desired thermal dose in this study would be less than that required to achieve

115

100% tumor cell kill; however, the main goal was to establish safety for heating breast carcinomas at therapeutic temperatures above 43°C with the adaptive phased array thermotherapy technology while demonstrating a tumor response in the form of tumor shrinkage or tumor cell kill.

6.2 PATIENTS, MATERIALS, AND METHODS

During the period of December 1999 to July 2000, 10 female patients with biopsy-proven breast carcinomas were enrolled in this Phase I study and treated with an FDA–Investigational Device Exemption–approved focused 915-MHz (megahertz) microwave adaptive phased array thermotherapy system (Microfocus APA 1000, Celsion [Canada] Limited, Ontario, Canada). This treatment system (refer to detailed discussion of the system in Chapter 3) produces a focused microwave field in the breast that is intended to heat and destroy high-water-, high-ion-content malignant breast tumors and microscopic carcinomas in the tumor margins. Patients were enrolled in the study provided that the tumor was at least 1 cm beneath the skin surface and not attached to the chest wall. Patients received breast thermotherapy treatment at Columbia Hospital in West Palm Beach, Florida, and at Harbor-UCLA Medical Center in Torrance, California. This Phase I study was approved and monitored by the Human Subjects Committee at each participating institution.

As shown in Figures 3.2 and 3.3 in Chapter 3, two air-cooled phase-controlled microwave waveguide applicators[2] were used to heat the breast carcinoma with the breast compressed (cranial-caudal) in the prone position similar to the positioning for stereo-tactic breast needle biopsy procedures.[3] A photograph of the Phase I breast thermotherapy treatment bed with dual-opposing microwave applicators is shown in **Figure 6.1**. This Phase I treatment bed had a fixed position, whereas the applicators were adjustable and could be positioned to the desired orientation facing the breast.

In this study, individual microwave and thermocouple probe sensors were placed within 16-gauge closed-end plastic catheters that were positioned under ultrasound (US) guidance to adaptively focus the microwave energy at the tumor and to measure the tumor temperature during thermotherapy. The needle (probe) sensor position-

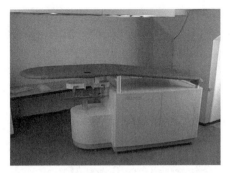

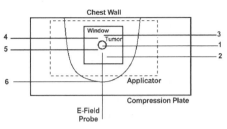

Figure 6.1   Phase I breast thermotherapy treatment bed with dual-opposing focused microwave applicators.

Source: Photo courtesy of Celsion (Canada), Limited.

Figure 6.2   Diagram showing the projective-view geometry of a parallel-opposed breast compression plate, ultra-sound window, microwave applicator (dashed rectangle), and probes used in the Phase I patient treatments.

Source: Gardner et al, Focused microwave phased array thermotherapy for primary breast cancer. *Annals Surg Oncol.* 2002;9(4):326–332.

ing in the breast is depicted in **Figure 6.2**. The microwave E-field focusing probe was positioned parallel to the polarization of the waveguide applicators to properly measure the focal field. The tumor thermocouple sensor (sensor 1), which was metallic, was positioned perpendicular to the polarization of the waveguide applicators so as not to perturb the microwave field.

The planned delivery of cumulative equivalent thermal dose of 60 minutes relative to 43°C (or a maximum treatment time of 40 minutes) to the tumor was the goal in each treatment. Target tumor temperatures desired in this study were in the range of 45° to 47°C. Five thermocouple sensors were taped to the skin (sensors 2 and 4 were caudal, sensors 3 and 5 were cranial) and nipple (sensor 6) to monitor the surface temperatures. To assess efficacy, imaging data based on mammography, US, magnetic resonance imaging, and pathology data were gathered before and after thermotherapy.

The total thermal dose in the tumor was computed in real time and displayed on the computer monitor during the treatment. The treatment was completed when the desired thermal dose was delivered to the tumor or the maximum treatment time (40 minutes) was reached. To determine the effectiveness of the treatment (tumor size reduction and tumor damage), US imaging with the patient supine and the breast and breast tumor of each patient in a consistent orientation was performed by a US technician before and after the microwave thermotherapy was administered, and pathology from needle core biopsy (single sample) and posttreatment mastectomy tissue was used to estimate tumor cell kill. One-dimensional tumor shrinkage was computed using $(1 - D_{final} \div D_{initial}) \times 100\%$, where D_{final} was the tumor diameter prior to surgery and $D_{initial}$ was the tumor diameter prior to thermotherapy. Tumor cell kill based on necrosis was estimated from hematoxylin and eosin pathology performed at each participating institution. M30 immunohistochemistry performed by IMPATH Inc. (Los Angeles, California) afforded a way to study efficacy of the treatment in tumor cells in terms of apoptosis-induced cell death. M30 staining characteristics in the pre- and postthermotherapy tumor tissue were compared. Care was taken to avoid any areas of obvious necrosis when comparing results. The M30 IgG2b monoclonal antibody (Roche Molecular Biochemicals, Indianapolis, Indiana) binds to a caspase-cleaved, formalin-resistant epitope of the cytokeratin-18 (CK-18) cytoskeletal produced during early apoptosis. The CK-18 molecule is a structural protein present in all epithelial cells. Prior studies in human carcinomas have shown that the M30 antibody reliably detects apoptosis when compared to the Terminal deoxynucleotidyl Transfer-mediated dUTP nick end labeling (TUNEL) and annexin V assays.[4]

Tumor cell kill based on M30 tests was calculated by first equating the prethermotherapy ratio of the percentage of cells staining positive and cells not staining to the ratio of the postthermotherapy positive-staining cells and the expected percentage of cells not staining if there was no thermotherapy treatment (denoted by the variable x). Solving for the variable x, the percentage of tumor cell kill is calculated by subtracting x from the percentage of cells not staining, and then normalizing this quantity by dividing by the percentage of cells not staining. For example, if B is the percentage of cells staining before thermotherapy and A is the percentage of cells staining after thermotherapy and lumpectomy, then it follows that $x = A(100 - B) \div B$, and the percentage of cell kill, denoted K, resulting from thermotherapy is expressed as

$$K = [(100 - A) - x] \div (100 - A) \qquad (6.1)$$

The total or cumulative equivalent minutes (CEM) thermal dose relative to 43°C was calculated from the measured temperature recorded by the thermocouple sensor in the tumor—the desired tumor thermal dose for this study was $CEM_{43°C} = 60$ minutes. The cumulative equivalent minutes thermal dose was also calculated for the surface sensor measurement positions.

Patients scheduled for mastectomy who met all the eligibility criteria and desired to participate in the microwave thermotherapy study were thoroughly instructed about its risks and benefits. After the consent form was signed, all the appropriate preoperative studies, tests, and measurements were made. The microwave thermotherapy was scheduled approximately 1 to 3 weeks before surgery. Data collected during the treatment were equipment performance, tumor and skin temperatures, and side effects. A 72-hour posttreatment information assessment was also collected. Based on physician assessment, other follow-ups were scheduled until surgery was performed. After surgery, the patients were seen as per recommended postsurgical follow-up periods.

6.3 PHASE I STUDY RESULTS

Ten patients in the Phase I study ranging in age from 43 to 82 years (mean 58.5 years) with breast carcinomas ranging in size from 0.9 to 8 cm (mean 4.2 cm, maximum dimension based on clinical exam) received focused microwave phased array thermotherapy (**Table 6.1**). In this study, 9 patients had invasive breast carcinomas and 1 patient had ductal carcinoma in situ only. All patients completed the thermotherapy treatment. In these treatments, the breast tissue compression thickness ranged from 4.5 to 6.5 cm (mean 5.6 cm). The peak tumor temperature, thermal dose to tumor and skin, tumor size reduction based on ultrasound, and tumor cell kill based on pathology are summarized in **Tables 6.2** and **6.3**.

In Table 6.2, the measured tumor thermal dose ranged from 24.5 to 100 equivalent minutes (mean 52 minutes) and the measured peak surface thermal dose ranged from 0 to 4.4 minutes (mean 0.8 minutes)—5 of 10 (50%) of patients received the desired thermal dose of

Table 6.1   Phase I Patient Demographics

Patient	Age (years)	Tumor Size* (cm)		Histology	Nuclear
		Clinical Exam	Ultrasound		
1	67	3.0	2.4	IDC	II
2	57	8.0	4.0	IDC	III
3	60	4.5	2.7	IDC	III
4	82	4.0	1.1	DCIS	N/A
5	48	2.5	1.9	IDC	II
6	52	5.0	2.9	IDC	III
7	75	5.0	1.5	IDC	II
8	47	0.9	0.9	IDC	II
9	54	3.5	1.1	IDC	II
10	43	5.5	3.4	IDC	II

*Maximal lesion diameter.
IDC = infiltrating ductal carcinoma, DCIS = ductal carcinoma in situ, N/A = Not Applicable

Source: Gardner RA, Vargas HI, Block JB, et al. Focused microwave phased array thermotherapy for primary breast cancer. *Ann Surg Oncol.* 2002;9(4):326–332.

Table 6.2   Phase I Focused Microwave Breast Thermotherapy Parameter Results

Patient	Tumor Size* (cm)		Peak Temperature (°C)		Thermal Dose (minutes)	
	Clinical Exam	Ultrasound	Tumor	Surface	Tumor	Surface
1	3.0	2.4	44.5	42.0	41.0	0.56
2	8.0	4.0	43.3	42.1	24.5	4.41
3	4.5	2.7	45.1	41.6	67.1	2.40
4	4.0	1.1	44.6	40.3	47.8	0.20
5	2.5	1.9	45.0	40.9	42.0	0.19
6	5.0	2.9	45.1	37.2	61.0	0.00
7	5.0	1.5	47.7	41.6	100.0	0.00
8	0.9	0.9	NM	41.7	NM	0.06
9	3.5	1.1	46.5	39.8	63.7	0.06
10	5.5	3.4	46.1	39.7	61.7	0.10

*Maximal lesion diameter.
NM = not measured.

Source: Gardner RA, Vargas HI, Block JB, et al. Focused microwave phased array thermotherapy for primary breast cancer. *Ann Surg Oncol.* 2002;9(4):326–332.

Table 6.3 Phase I Breast Carcinoma Response for a Single Focused
Microwave Thermotherapy Dose

Patient	Time to Surgery (days)	% Tumor Size Reduction (Ultrasound)	% Tumor Cell Kill	
			Necrosis	Apoptosis
1	7	29	0	97.2
2	8	60	0	0.0
3	7	29	60	81.7
4	6	0	0	NM
5	5	0	0	NM
6	15	42	0	89.2
7	13	0	40	0.0
8	27	29	0	92.7
9	18	0	50	83.5
10	13	59	40	93.8

NM = not measured.

Source: Gardner RA, Vargas HI, Block JB, et al. Focused microwave phased array thermotherapy for primary breast cancer. *Ann Surg Oncol.* 2002;9(4):326–332.

60 equivalent minutes. The microwave treatment time ranged from 12 to 40 minutes (mean 34.7 minutes). During each treatment, the tumor temperature was raised significantly higher than that of the skin and nipple. Peak tumor temperature ranged from 43.3° to 47.7°C (mean 45.3°C) and the peak surface temperature for all sensors ranged from 37.2° to 42.1°C (mean 40.7°C); thus, the mean peak tumor temperature achieved was 4.2°C higher than the mean peak surface temperature. The measured tumor and peak surface temperature and power during treatment for Patient 9 are shown in **Figure 6.3**—for this patient, the initial tumor temperature was 33.8°C, the heating rate was approximately 0.4°C/minute, the peak tumor temperature reached was 46.5°C, and the peak skin temperature was only 39.8°C.

As shown in Table 6.3, the thermotherapy treatments achieved evidence of tumor size reduction in six patients and tumor necrosis in four patients—8 of the 10 patients treated with thermotherapy responded with either tumor shrinkage or tumor necrosis. Apoptosis analysis was performed on the excised tissue for the 8 of 10 tumors that responded to thermotherapy. From M30 immunohistochemistry, it was found in 6 out of the 8 responding tumors that there was a

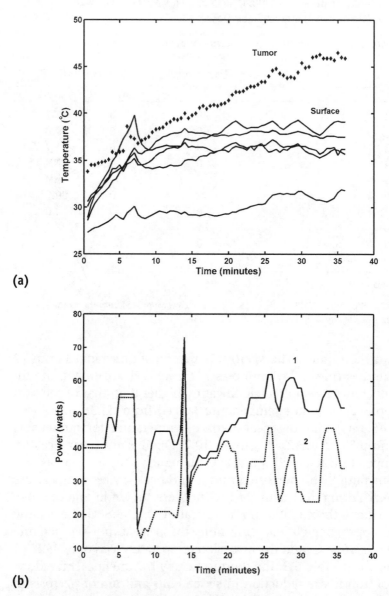

(a)

(b)

Figure 6.3 **(a)** Measured temperature in tumor and peak surface temperature during focused microwave phased array thermotherapy treatment for Patient #9 in the Phase I clinical study. **(b)** Microwave power for the two channels during thermotherapy.

significant decrease in staining of the thermotherapy-treated tumor cells. Prior to thermotherapy, from the biopsy specimen, the percentage of tumor cells staining M30-positive ranged from 70% to 90% (mean 81.7%, standard deviation 9.8%). After thermotherapy and lumpectomy, the percentage of tumor cells staining M30-positive ranged from 20% to 60% (mean 31.7%, standard deviation 16%). The decreased postthermotherapy staining observed when compared with the pretreated tumor is likely related to a nonviable cellular stage beyond the detection of the M30 antibody. These observations should be corroborated with other complementary apoptosis stains (such as TUNEL), which detect cellular products in later stages of apoptosis.[4] Of the 8 patients that responded with either tumor shrinkage or tumor necrosis, apoptosis-based cell kill was calculated from the pre- and postthermotherapy M30 stains and showed in 6 patients between 82% and 97% tumor cell kill (mean 89.7%) in the cells that did not stain M30-positive.

Side effects and their presumed cause in this study were as follows. In the first three patients, only two auxiliary fans surrounding the breast were used to cool the skin and nipple and peak surface temperatures of 41.9°C (mean) occurred (at the upper limit of 42°C desired) and peak surface thermal dose 2.5 minutes (mean) occurred. In the subsequent patient treatments, up to four auxiliary fans cooled the skin and nipple, which may have helped reduce the peak temperature (mean 40.2°C) and thermal dose (mean 0.09 minute) in the surface tissues for Patients 4 to 10. Limited (range 0.6 × 1.5 cm to 1.2 × 3.5 cm) flap necrosis occurred in the first three patients and may have been caused by the combination of thin skin flaps, the peak skin temperature, skin thermal dose, and the short time (7 to 8 days) between thermotherapy and mastectomy. The first three patients ranged in age from 57 to 67 years (mean 64.3 years), and the subsequent seven patients ranged in age from 43 to 82 years (mean 57.3 years). Because the difference in mean age between the first three patients and the last seven is only 10%, patient age does not appear to be a significant parameter for flap necrosis in this study. Additionally, both prethermotherapy tumor size (based on US measurements) and tumor grade did not correlate with flap necrosis. As a result of thermotherapy for Patient 3, a small blister (approximately 1-cm diameter) occurred, which healed completely with no treatment required and presented no special considerations during surgery.

6.4 DISCUSSION OF PHASE I STUDY

This Phase I study demonstrates that a significant thermal dose (mean $CEM_{43°C}$ = 52 minutes) can be delivered to breast carcinomas at central depth with reduced superficial thermal dose (mean $CEM_{43°C}$ = 0.8 minute). In the 10 treatments, peak tumor temperature ranged from 43.3° to 47.7°C, and peak surface temperatures ranged from 37.2° to 42.1°C. To determine the effectiveness of the heat-alone thermotherapy, the results of imaging and pathology data were analyzed. Tumor size reduction ranging from 29% to 60% (mean 41%) occurred in 18 days or less in 6 out of 10 patients (60%) based on US measurements. Postthermotherapy (27 days or less) mastectomy specimens showed that, in 4 out of the 10 treatments (40%), significant tumor necrosis estimated at 40% to 60% (mean 48%) of total tumor volume occurred, and that in 6 of 8 patients tumor cell kill estimated at 82% to 97% (mean 89.7%) based on apoptosis measurements occurred. It is possible that a longer observation time after thermotherapy could have resulted in further tumor size reduction and increased tumor cell kill.

The pathology data of this study suggest that achieving a 60-minute thermal dose and peak temperature $> 45°C$ is correlated with the onset of significant tumor necrosis, and that a higher dose and peak temperature are required for increased tumor necrosis for breast carcinomas. Significant apoptosis-based cell kill occurred for peak tumor temperatures in the range of 44° to 46.5°C with thermal dose in the range of $CEM_{43°C}$ 40 to 67 minutes. Similar results are observed for in vitro thermotherapy studies in murine mastocytoma, demonstrating that cell death is a result of apoptosis for temperatures in the range of 43° to 45°C and is a result of necrosis for temperatures of 45° to 47°C when heat is applied for 30 minutes.[5] The two patients (Patients 4 and 5) for which thermotherapy had no size reduction or necrosis effect on the tumor, received less than 60 minutes equivalent thermal dose and had peak tumor temperatures not greater than 45°C. Patients 4 and 5 had surgery after thermotherapy within the shortest period of time (6 and 5 days, respectively). It is possible that waiting a longer period of time following thermotherapy would have resulted in some tumor response for these two patients.

6.5 SUMMARY

In Phase I tests of a clinical focused microwave phased array thermotherapy system, 10 patients have been treated and a significant thermal dose was delivered to breast carcinomas 1 to 8 cm in maximum clinical dimension and located at central depth in the compressed breast. Eight of 10 patients (80%) had a tumor response based on tumor shrinkage measured by US or tumor cell kill based on necrosis and apoptosis measurements. A higher tumor thermal dose than that used in this study, or more than one heat treatment, would be required to attempt complete pathologic tumor cell kill. The monoclonal antibody used in this study provided primarily a weak positive stain for early apoptosis—other antibodies could be investigated in future studies to provide a stronger stain and more accurately estimate the percentage of tumor cell kill based on apoptosis-associated cell death. Focused microwave phased array thermotherapy is promising based on these Phase I results. Phase II efficacy studies at increased thermal dose in a larger group of breast cancer patients have recently been conducted and are described in the next chapter.

REFERENCES

1. Gardner RA, Vargas HI, Block JB, Vogel CL, Fenn AJ, Kuehl GV, Doval M. Focused microwave phased array thermotherapy for primary breast cancer. *Ann Surg Oncol.* 2002;9(4):326–332.
2. Cheung AY, Dao T, Robinson JE. Dual beam TEM applicator for direct contact heating of dielectrically encapsulated malignant mouse tumor. *Radio Science.* 1977;12(6(S)suppl):81–85.
3. Bassett L, Winchester DP, Caplan, RB, et al. Stereotactic core needle biopsy of the breast: a report of the Joint Task Force of the American College of Radiology, American College of Surgeons, and College of American Pathologists. *CA Cancer J Clin.* 1997;17:171–190.
4. Leers MPG, Kolgen W, Bjorklund V, et al. Immunocytochemical detection and mapping of a cytokeratin 18 neo-epitope exposed during early apoptosis. *J Pathol.* 1999;187:567–572.
5. Harmon BV, Corder AM, Colins RJ, et al. Cell death induced in a murine mastocytoma by 42–47°C heating *in vitro:* evidence that the form of death changes from apoptosis to necrosis above a critical heat load. *Int J Radiat Biol.* 1990;58:854–858.

Phase II Thermal Dose Escalation Study for Early-Stage Breast Carcinomas in Patients Scheduled for Breast Conservation Surgery

7.1 INTRODUCTION

As described in Chapter 6, a 10-patient Phase I safety study[1] of preoperative thermotherapy using externally applied focused microwaves for treatment of primary breast cancer demonstrated that tumor temperatures in the range of 45.1° to 47.7°C and tumor thermal doses in the range of $CEM_{43°C}$ 25 to 103 equivalent minutes (relative to 43°C) produced breast tumor necrosis ranging from 40% to 60% in 4 of 10 (40%) of patients. Tumor response in the form of necrosis, apoptosis, or tumor shrinkage occurred in 8 of 10 (80%) of patients.

The Phase I results indicate that higher temperatures and higher thermal doses are required for increased breast tumor response. For the tumor temperatures and thermal doses administered, this result of incomplete tumor necrosis for the Phase I study is consistent with the in vitro results presented in Chapter 2, Figure 2.1. To investigate an increased tumor response based on pathologically measured necrosis, a Phase II study was designed to establish the safety, feasibility, and efficacy of preoperative focused microwave phased array (FMPA) thermotherapy at increasing thermal dose in patients with early-stage T1, T2 infiltrating ductal or lobular carcinoma (invasive breast cancer).[2] Patients treated under this Food and Drug Administration (FDA)–approved Phase II study were patients scheduled for wide-excision lumpectomy and radiation therapy for breast conservation.

7.2 PATIENTS, MATERIALS, AND METHODS

7.2.1 Patient Selection

Between May 2001 and July 2002, patients with invasive breast carcinoma seen at Harbor-UCLA Medical Center in Torrance, California; the University of Oklahoma in Oklahoma City, Oklahoma; Columbia Hospital in West Palm Beach, Florida; and Martin-Luther University in Hale, Germany, were invited to participate in this FDA-approved thermal dose-escalation safety and efficacy clinical trial. This study was approved and monitored by the Human Subjects Committee at each participating institution. Other patient eligibility criteria included (1) Karnofski score >70%, (2) core-needle-biopsy-proven invasive breast cancer, (3) breast conservation treatment was planned, (4) the tumor had to be visible and measurable by ultrasound, (5) the absence of involvement of the skin or pectoralis muscle. All patients were required to undergo counseling and to sign a written informed consent document.

Specific exclusion criteria were pregnancy, breast-feeding, and presence of breast implants, pacemakers or defibrillators. Other exclusion criteria were (1) known bleeding diathesis, (2) laboratory evidence of coagulopathy (prothrombin time, international normalized ratio >1.5; partial prothrombin time >1.5), (3) thrombocytopenia (platelet count < 100,000/mm3), (4) anticoagulant therapy, or (5) evidence of chronic liver disease or renal failure.

7.2.2 Study Design and Treatment Plan

This Phase II study was designed as a prospective, multicenter, non-randomized, dose-escalation study. Focused microwave treatment was performed with the patient in prone position on an outpatient basis using local anesthesia in the treated breast. An FDA–Investigational Device Exemption–approved two-channel 915-MHz (megahertz) focused microwave adaptive phased array thermotherapy system (Microfocus-1000 APA, Celsion [Canada] Limited, Ontario Canada) was used in this study. A photograph of the breast thermotherapy treatment system is shown in Chapter 3, Figure 3.4.

This treatment system produces a focused microwave field in the breast to heat and destroy high-water-content tumor tissue. The clinical rationale for this approach of focused microwave phased array FMPA thermotherapy for thermal ablation of early-stage breast carcinomas is described in Chapters 1 and 2. Patients were monitored for toxicity following each treatment. In this study, a combination E-field sensor and fiber-optic temperature probe were inserted in a single catheter (16-gauge Flexineedle sharp end plastic catheter, Best Medical) with the tip of the catheter in the approximate center of the breast tumor. A photograph of the combination E-field and fiber-optic temperature sensor is shown in Chapter 3, Figure 3.5. Seven thermocouple sensors monitored the skin and nipple temperature as depicted in Chapter 3, Figure 3.6.

As discussed in Section 4.5, experimental studies support the concept that tumor cell heating for 60 minutes at 43°C is tumoricidal, and the period of time to kill tumor cells decreases by a factor of two for each degree increase in temperature above about 43°C. Thus, the treatment time required for a 120-minute treatment at 43°C can be reduced to about 3.75 minutes at 48°C, which is referred to as equivalent thermal dose ($CEM_{43°C}$, cumulative equivalent minutes relative to 43°C). The CEM thermal dose was calculated from the measured temperatures recorded by the sensors in the tumor and on the skin—the desired tumor thermal dose during microwave heating for this study was in the range of 80 to 120 $CEM_{43°C}$. Once the desired thermal dose is achieved, the microwave power is reduced to zero and breast compression is maintained during a 5-minute cooldown period. During this period, because of the thermal insulation of the surrounding breast tissues, the thermal dose continues to accumulate in the tumor; however, the surface temperatures drop to normal values very quickly.

Escalation of thermal dose was performed in groups of five patients at progressively increasing doses of 80 CEM, 100 CEM, and 120 CEM plus additional equivalent minutes during the 5-minute cooldown. Treatment of an additional 10 patients at the highest dose was planned if no dose-limiting toxicity was reached. If a patient did not complete the planned thermal dose in the first treatment, an optional second thermotherapy treatment could be administered to achieve the planned (cumulative) thermal dose. All toxicities were graded and reported according to dose level, and toxicities were assessed after therapy. Breast surgery was planned to be performed no later than 60 days after the administration of thermotherapy.

Tumor cell kill was based on tumor necrosis and was estimated from Hematoxylin and Eosin stained histological sections from wide local excision of the primary breast tumor. Necrosis was estimated and expressed as a percentage of necrotic tumor areas in relation to necrotic and viable tumor areas.

Adverse events, vital signs, and laboratory measurements (complete blood count, blood urea nitrogen and creatinine, bilirubin, serum glutamic-oxaloacetic transaminase, serum glutamic-pyruvic transaminase, alkaline phosphatase, and routine chemistries) were monitored to evaluate the safety and tolerability of the thermal dose. Performance status was recorded after thermal therapy.

7.2.3 Statistical Analysis

A model to compute the percentage of tumor necrosis as a function of either tumor thermal dose or peak tumor temperature achieved was developed based on linear regression to determine the best fit to the measured data.[3] With this linear regression model, a straight line is determined that minimizes the sum of the squares of the difference between the model tumor necrosis and measured tumor necrosis data.

7.3 PHASE II STUDY RESULTS

Twenty-five patients were included in this study. Patient demographics and tumor characteristics are summarized in **Table 7.1**. Mean patient age was 57.2 years (range 38 to 72 years). At enrollment, the mean tumor diameter based on ultrasound was 1.76 cm (range 0.7 to 2.8 cm). Twenty-four of 25 (96%) patients tolerated and completed the thermotherapy treatment.

A photograph of a patient receiving focused microwave breast thermotherapy is shown in **Figure 7.1**. In this photograph, the patient is prone, the breast is compressed, and the air-cooling tubes are directed at the breast to cool the surface with room-temperature air. For this particular treatment, the breast compression was medial lateral.

Tumor and surface temperature measurements for an example treatment are depicted in **Figure 7.2(a)**, and **Figure 7.2(b)** shows the corresponding commanded microwave power during this treatment. In Figure 7.2(a), the initial tumor temperature at the start of treatment was 40.7°C. The microwave heating period was 14.5 minutes and the peak

Table 7.1 Demographics and Tumor Characteristics of the Phase II Study Population

N		25
Age	Mean, years	57.2
	Range, years	38–72
Tumor diameter	Mean, cm	1.76
(ultrasound)	Range, cm	0.7–2.8
Histology	Invasive ductal	80%
	Invasive lobular	8%
	Colloid	8%
	Other	4%
Tumor Grade	High Grade	25%
	Intermediate Grade	56%
	Low Grade	19%

Source: Vargas HI, Dooley WC, Gardner RA, et al. Focused microwave phased array thermotherapy for ablation of early-stage breast cancer: results of thermal dose escalation. *Ann Surg Oncol.* 2004;11(2):139–146. With kind permission of Springer Science and Business Media.

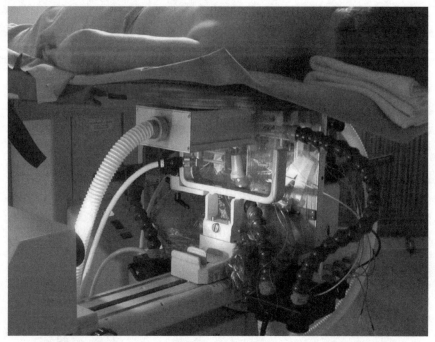

Figure 7.1   Phase II breast cancer patient receiving focused microwave breast thermotherapy treatment. (Photo courtesy of Celsion [Canada] Limited)

tumor temperature achieved was 48.1°C. The peak surface temperature for all the surface sensors was 36.3°C during this treatment. Once the microwave power was turned off, the skin temperatures dropped rapidly (exponentially) to pretreatment temperatures while, as a result of thermal insulation and breast compression, the tumor temperature dropped slowly and nearly linearly at approximately 1.3°C/minute and continued to accumulate thermal dose. The linear drop in temperature is characteristic of phantom-like nonperfused tissues.

In this study, tumoricidal temperatures ($>43°C$) were reached in 23 patients (92%). The breast tissue compression thickness ranged from 3.5 to 6.5 cm and was adjusted during microwave thermotherapy as necessary to maintain patient comfort. Patients underwent breast-conserving surgery on average 17 days after thermotherapy (range: 6–38 days).

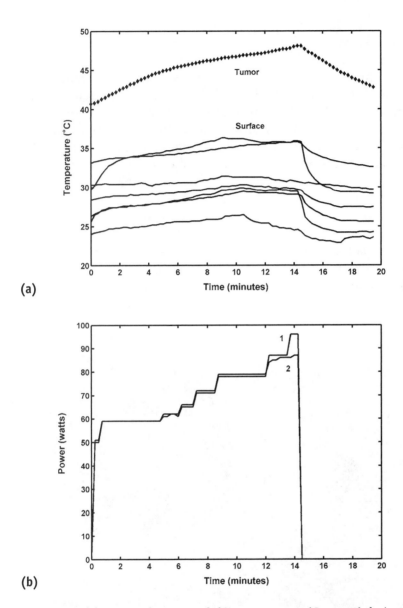

Figure 7.2 (a) Measured tumor and skin temperatures (Case #19) during focused microwave phased array thermotherapy treatment of breast cancer in the intact breast during the Phase II clinical study. (b) Microwave power for the two channels during thermotherapy.

There was evidence of pathologic necrosis in 17 of 25 (68%) patients. An example of the gross tumor necrosis induced by microwave thermal therapy for case 15 is depicted in **Figure 7.3**—in this case, the tumor necrosis was 85%, the peak tumor temperature was 48.4°C, and the equivalent thermal dose was 206 minutes. There was complete (100%) ablation of invasive carcinoma in two cases; however, both patients had residual in-situ breast cancer. There was one additional patient with a single cluster of residual tumor cells (tumor necrosis estimated at 99.9%). The extent of necrosis in the other cases ranged from 25% to 90%. Tumor-free margins with breast conservation surgery were obtained in 24 (96%) patients. Histologic tumor response in the three cohorts of patients according to planned thermal dose is depicted in **Table 7.2**.

Six of 25 subjects were excluded from analysis of the efficacy of thermal energy in inducing pathologic necrosis as a result of inaccurate tumor temperature recordings (4 cases) and delivery of suboptimal thermal dose (2 cases). Data for the 19 included patients are

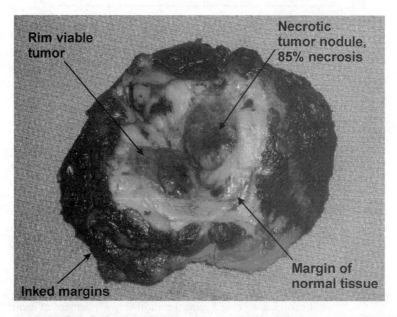

Figure 7.3   Photograph of gross section in which focused microwave thermotherapy induced 85% tumor necrosis for Case #15 in the Phase II study.

Source: Vargas HI, Dooley WC, Gardner RA, et al. Focused microwave phased array thermotherapy for ablation of early-stage breast cancer: results of thermal dose escalation. *Ann Surg Oncol.* 2004;11(2):139–146. With kind permission of Springer Science and Business Media.

Table 7.2 Histologic Tumor Response in the Three Groups of Phase II
Focused Microwave Thermotherapy Patients According to
Planned Thermal Dose

CEM	N	Pathologic Necrosis (%)
80	Single treatment (N = 3)	0, 0, 0
	Two treatments (N = 2)	80, 85
100	Single treatment	
	(N = 5)	0, 50, 70 ,70, 95
120	Single treatment	0, 0, 0, 0, 25, 50, 50, 60
	(N = 15)	80, 85, 85, 90, 99.9, 100, 100

CEM, cumulative equivalent minutes.

Source: Vargas HI, Dooley WC, Gardner RA, et al. Focused microwave phased array thermotherapy
for ablation of early-stage breast cancer: results of thermal dose escalation. *Ann Surg Oncol.*
2004;11(2):139–146. With kind permission of Springer Science and Business Media.

shown in **Table 7.3**. Eight patients received a cumulative thermal
dose in the range of 158.9 to 206 minutes, and all had significant tumor necrosis (range 60% to 100%, mean 84%). Nine patients received a thermal dose in the range of 107.8 to 147.8 minutes and 6
of 9 (67%) had tumor necrosis (range 25% to 95%, mean 40%). Two
patients received a thermal dose in the range of 82.8 to 97.2 minutes,
and 1 of 2 (50%) had tumor necrosis (range 0% to 50%, mean 25%).
Fourteen of 15 patients (93.3%) receiving a peak tumor temperature
$\geq 46.9\,^{\circ}$C had tumor necrosis (range 25% to 100%, mean 72.1%).

Linear regression was performed to predict tumor response based
on thermal dose and peak temperature achieved. The percentage of tumor necrosis in relation to the thermal dose is expressed graphically
in **Figure 7.4**. A thermal dose of 140 $CEM_{43^\circ C}$ is predictive of a 50%
tumor response, and 210 CEM is predictive of a 100% tumor response
($P = 0.003$). The percentage of tumor necrosis in relation to the peak
tumor temperature is displayed in **Figure 7.5**. The univariate linear regression model predicts that a peak tumor temperature of 47.4°C is
predictive of a 50% tumor response and a peak tumor temperature of
49.7°C is predictive of a 100% tumor response ($P = 0.01$). The predicted thermal dose and peak tumor temperature for 0%, 50%, 85%,
and 100% necrosis are summarized in **Table 7.4**. Both peak tumor
temperature and thermal dose show statistically significant association with tumor necrosis. Thermal dose is the better predictor of tumor necrosis. Using a multivariate regression model containing both

Table 7.3   Treatment Results Listed by Increasing Cumulative Thermal Dose and Percentage of Tumor Necrosis by Tumor Volume from the Phase II Study

Case	Number of Treatments	Thermal Dose $CEM_{43°C}$	Peak Tumor Temperature (°C)	Tumor Necrosis (%)
5	1	82.8	45.9	0
6	1	97.2	47.0	50
9	1	107.8	47.3	70
8	1	116.5	45.9	70
10	1	116.7	47.4	95
3	1	122.0	45	0
23	1	124.3	45.9	0
24	1	136.9	47.3	50
13	1	137.8	47.0	25
17	1	142.0	47.5	0
22	1	147.8	47.7	50
21	1	158.9	47.8	100
11	1	166.8	48.3	60
20	1	169.6	50	85
4	2	175.5	46.9	85
12	1	175.8	48	80
19	1	180.0	48.1	99.9
1	2	183.9	46.9	75
15	1	206.0	48.4	85

Note: These 19 cases were used in efficacy analysis. In this group, a tumoricidal temperature (43°C) was reached and temperature recordings were accurate.

CEM, cumulative equivalent minutes.

Source: Vargas HI, Dooley WC, Gardner RA, et al. Focused microwave phased array thermotherapy for ablation of early-stage breast cancer: results of thermal dose escalation. *Ann Surg Oncol.* 2004;11(2):139–146. With kind permission of Springer Science and Business Media.

Table 7.4   Projected Thermal Dose and Peak Tumor Temperature Required for Necrosis of Invasive Breast Carcinomas

Tumor Necrosis (%)	Thermal Dose $CEM_{43°C}$	Peak Tumor Temperature (°C)
0	<71	>44.5
55	140.3	47.1
85	188.9	49.0
100	>209.8	>49.7

CEM, cumulative equivalent minutes.

Source: Vargas HI, Dooley WC, Gardner RA, et al. Focused microwave phased array thermotherapy for ablation of early-stage breast cancer: results of thermal dose escalation. *Ann Surg Oncol.* 2004;11(2):139–146. With kind permission of Springer Science and Business Media.

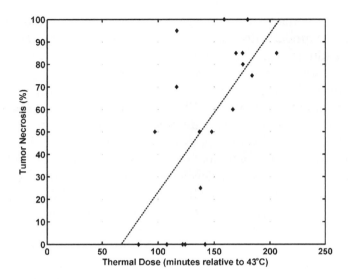

Figure 7.4 Pathologic tumor necrosis (*N*) in relation to tumor thermal dose (CEM) dose for 19 patients. The dashed line is the linear regression fit (*N* = 0.719 CEM − 50.902) to the experimental data.

Source: Vargas HI, Dooley WC, Gardner RA, et al. Focused microwave phased array thermotherapy for ablation of early-stage breast cancer: results of thermal dose escalation. *Ann Surg Oncol.* 2004;11(2):139–146. With kind permission of Springer Science and Business Media.

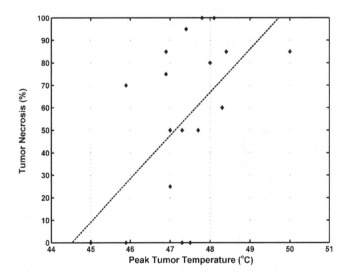

Figure 7.5 Pathologic tumor necrosis (*N*) in relation to tumor peak tempertature (*T*ₚ) for 19 patients. The dashed line is the linear regression fit (*N* = 19.128 *T*ₚ − 851.176) to the experimental data.

Source: Vargas HI, Dooley WC, Gardner RA, et al. Focused microwave phased array thermotherapy for ablation of early-stage breast cancer: results of thermal dose escalation. *Ann Surg Oncol.* 2004;11(2):139–146. With kind permission of Springer Science and Business Media.

independent variables does not significantly improve the predictive power of the model. This is a result in large part of the correlation between the tumor peak temperature and thermal dose treatment parameters (Spearman correlation $r = 0.77$, $P < 0.0001$).

Side effects in this study were as follows. In the first group of 5 patients scheduled to receive 80 CEM, 3 patients had one treatment and 2 patients were given two treatments. Thermotherapy was well tolerated. Short-lived erythema developed in the skin of the treated breast in 2 of 5 (40%) patients. In patients assigned to the 100 CEM thermal dose, 3 of 5 (60%) developed short-lived erythema, 2 of 5 (40%) experienced mild pain during treatment, and 1 of 5 (20%) developed a first-degree burn of the treated skin that completely healed and presented no special considerations during surgery.

In the last group of patients, scheduled to receive 120 CEM, one patient reported severe pain in the first 4 minutes of thermotherapy and the treatment was stopped—the highest skin temperature was 37.2°C and the tumor temperature was 39.2°C at the time the microwave energy was turned off. Seven of 15 (47%) experienced pain, 4 of 15 (27%) developed short-lived skin erythema, 5 of 15 (33%) developed edema of the breast or areola, and 2 of 15 (13%) patients developed skin thermal burns (first-degree and third-degree). The third-degree burn occurred over a small area (8-mm diameter) enclosing the focusing probe skin entry point, which was within the microwave field in proximity to one of the microwave applicators.

7.4 DISCUSSION OF PHASE II STUDY

The objective of using minimally invasive treatment techniques is to cause complete local tumor regression and long-term local control of breast cancer with minimal damage to the surrounding normal breast tissue. Other characteristics of the ideal treatment are that it must be an outpatient procedure using a percutaneous or transcutaneous application without the need of sedation or general anesthesia. The morbidity and local complications must be minimal.

In this clinical trial, two-thirds of patients exhibited various degrees of coagulative necrosis that ranged from 25% to 100%. Complete ablation of invasive breast cancer was achieved in two cases, and there was only a residual cluster of cancer cells in one additional case. Success was achieved in the subset of patients receiving higher thermal doses. The main objective of this study of FMPA thermotherapy was to find the dose necessary to cause complete tumor ablation without clinically significant toxicity.

The thermal dose was escalated in 25 patients. This study has established that both thermal dose and peak temperature show statistically significant association with the presence of tumor necrosis in the wide local excision specimen. Based on this statistical model, 100% tumor cell death is expected when a minimum thermal dose of 209.8 $CEM_{43°C}$ and a peak tumor temperature of 49.7°C are achieved. Furthermore, the therapeutic window of FMPA thermotherapy takes place at a point where no significant toxicity is seen. Future studies conducted at therapeutic doses of FMPA thermotherapy will provide meaningful information regarding the success of this therapy based on pathological response. In practice, with transcutaneous focused microwaves it might be difficult to deliver temperatures of 49.7°C consistently to tumors, and a lower tumor temperature of about 48°C would always be easier to achieve. Based on the in vitro data presented in Section 2.2 and the discussion of equivalent thermal dose in Section 4.5, a thermal dose higher than about 256 to 288 $CEM_{43°C}$ might be required for consistent 100% tumor cell death if a target tumor temperature of 48°C is used.

In the current study, FMPA thermotherapy was conducted by the placement of a percutaneous sensor catheter for focusing of the microwaves (E-field sensor) and measurement of tumor temperatures (temperature sensor). Temperature sensor positioning was not extensively evaluated in this study. However, in two cases, large areas of necrosis secondary to FMPA thermotherapy were located eccentrically to the tumor mass. A residual area of viable tumor was then marginally missed because of imperfect targeting. Izzo,[4] based on experience with radiofrequency ablation, has recognized the importance of accurate placement of the percutaneous probe in the success of percutaneous tumor ablation. Accurate placement of the percutaneous probe is also required in focused microwave thermotherapy.

An observation arising from this study is the 4% rate of positive margins, in comparison to reported incidences of positive margins of 4% to 44% in the literature.[5-8] The two microwave applicators have rectangular apertures that face the compressed breast tissue.[9] The effective microwave radiation field encompasses an approximate 6-cm by 8-cm area in the breast tissue in a plane parallel to the compression plates. In the compressed breast thickness dimension, the effective microwave field extends approximately 1.5 cm on either side of the focal target point in the tumor. This microwave field distribution has the potential of creating a large volume of tumor cell kill. A hypothesis that requires critical study is the question of whether the use of thermotherapy treatment prior to breast conservation surgery provides significant tumor cell kill at the margins, is responsible for a low incidence of positive margins, and can contribute to a reduction in the need for reexcisions required compared to surgery alone.

7.5 SUMMARY

The Phase II results of preoperative focused microwave thermotherapy presented in this chapter indicate that thermotherapy induces breast tumor necrosis, and there is a threshold thermal dose of approximately 210 thermal equivalent minutes (relative to 43°C) that is predictive of 100% cell kill for breast cancer tumors. The next chapter investigates the use of preoperative focused microwave thermotherapy in a randomized setting to determine whether potential patient benefits such as reduced positive margins or reduced second incisions might be possible.

REFERENCES

1. Gardner RA, Vargas HI, Block JB, Vogel CL, Fenn AJ, Kuehl GV, Doval M. Focused microwave phased array thermotherapy for primary breast cancer. *Ann Surg Oncol.* 2002;9(4):326–332.

2. Vargas HI, Dooley WC, Gardner RA, Gonzalez KD, Venegas R, Heywang-Kobrunner SH, Fenn AJ. Focused microwave phased array thermotherapy for ablation of early-stage breast cancer: results of thermal dose escalation. *Ann Surg Oncol.* 2004;11(2):139–146.

3. Armitage P, Berry G. *Statistical Methods in Medical Research.* 3rd ed. Oxford, England: Blackwell Science; 1994:156–163, 283–311.

4. Izzo F, Thomas R, Delrio P, et al. Radiofrequency ablation in patients with primary breast carcinoma. A pilot study of 26 patients. *Cancer.* 2001;92: 2036–2044.

5. Recht A, Come SE, Henderson IC, et al. The sequencing of chemotherapy and radiation therapy after conservative surgery for early stage breast cancer. *N Engl J Med.* 1996;334:1356–1361.

6. Park CC, Mitsumori M, Nixon A, et al. Outcome at 8 years after breast-conserving surgery and radiation therapy for invasive breast cancer: influence of margin status and systemic therapy on local recurrence. *J Clin Oncol.* 2000;18: 1668–1675.

7. Smitt MC, Nowels KW, Zdeblick MJ. The importance of lumpectomy surgical margin status in long term results of breast conservation. *Cancer.* 1995;76: 259–267.

8. Ryoo MC, Kagan AT, Wollin M, et al. Prognostic factors for recurrence and cosmesis in 393 patients after radiation therapy for early mammary carcinoma. *Radiology.* 1989;172:555–559.

9. Fenn AJ, Wolf GL, Fogle RM. An adaptive phased array for targeted heating of deep tumors in intact breast: animal study results. *Int J Hyperthermia.* 1999;15(1):45–61.

Randomized Study of Focused Microwave Thermotherapy for Early-Stage Breast Carcinomas in Patients Scheduled for Breast Conservation Surgery: Thermotherapy Prior to Surgery Compared to Surgery Alone

CHAPTER

8

8.1 INTRODUCTION

The clinical rationale for the use of preoperative thermotherapy for early-stage invasive breast cancer is described in Chapter 1. The aim of the clinical study reviewed in this chapter was to verify the required minimum thermal dose (established from the results discussed in Chapter 7) to heat safely and kill primary breast carcinomas prior to surgery in a multicenter randomized setting, and to determine whether thermotherapy prior to surgery could reduce the rate of close or positive margins and/or the rate of second incision compared to surgery alone.[1] Tumor temperatures desired in this study were in the range of 48° to 52°C with the equivalent tumor thermal dose delivered (during active microwave heating) in the range of 140 to 180 minutes relative to 43°C while avoiding skin damage and other morbidity.

Based on the thermal dose escalation results[2] reviewed in Chapter 7, to reach the desired minimum thermal dose of 210 minutes (210 $CEM_{43°C}$), additional thermal equivalent minutes were accumulated during a cooldown phase after microwaves were powered off and the tumor temperature was reduced to baseline while the breast was maintained in compression.

8.2 PATIENTS, MATERIALS, AND METHODS

8.2.1 Patient Selection

Between November 2002 and May 2004, patients with primary invasive breast carcinomas (T1, T2) seen at (1) University of Oklahoma, Oklahoma City; (2) Harbor-UCLA Medical Center, Torrance, California; (3) Comprehensive Breast Center, Coral Springs, Florida; (4) Mroz-Baier Breast Care Center, Memphis, Tennessee; (5) Pearl Place, Tacoma, Washington; (6) St. Joseph's Hospital, Orange, California; (7) Royal Bolton Hospital, Bolton, United Kingdom; (8) Breast Care Specialists, Norfolk, Virginia; (9) Breast Care, Las Vegas, Nevada; and (10) Carolina Surgery, Gastonia, North Carolina, were invited to participate in this Food and Drug Administration (FDA)–approved thermal dose safety and efficacy clinical trial. This study was approved and monitored by the Human Subjects Committee at each participating institution. Other eligibility criteria included (1) Karnofski performance status > 70%, (2) core-needle-biopsy-proven invasive breast cancer, (3) planned breast conservation treatment by partial mastectomy or lumpectomy followed by radiation therapy, (4) visible tumor measurable by ultrasound, and (5) absence of involvement of the skin or pectoralis muscle. All patients were required to undergo counseling and to sign written informed consent forms.

Specific exclusion criteria were pregnancy, breast-feeding, and presence of breast implants, clinically significant heart disease, pacemakers or defibrillators, unable to tolerate prone position or breast compression, or diagnosis of cancer made by lumpectomy or incisional biopsy. Other exclusion criteria were: known bleeding diathesis, laboratory evidence of coagulopathy (prothrombin time, international normalized ratio ≥ 1.5; partial prothrombin ≥ 1.5), thrombocytopenia (platelet count $< 100,000/mm^3$), (4) anticoagulant therapy, (5) evidence of chronic liver disease or renal failure, (6) presence of any factor or condition, other than tumor size, that would preclude lumpectomy including multicentric disease or prior history of collagen vascular disease, or (7) breast cancer with a high probability of extensive intra-ductal in situ disease.

8.2.2 Study Design and Treatment Plan

This study was designed as a prospective, multicenter randomized study with two treatment arms (thermotherapy plus surgery, and surgery alone as the control arm). Microwave treatment was performed on an outpatient basis using local anesthesia with patients in the prone position. An FDA-approved two-channel 915-MHz (megahertz) focused microwave adaptive phased array thermotherapy system (Microfocus-1000 APA; Celsion [Canada] Limited), as discussed in Chapter 3, Section 3.2, was used in this study (see Figure 3.4). This minimally invasive treatment system produces a focused microwave field in the compressed breast to heat and destroy high-water-, high-ion-content tumor tissue. A 16-gauge (1.65-mm OD [outside diameter], 1.22-mm ID [inside diameter]) closed-end plastic catheter was inserted into the tumor under ultrasound guidance, and a single-use disposable combination E-field focusing sensor (1.12-mm OD) and temperature sensor (Figure 3.5) were inserted in the catheter to focus the microwaves and measure the tumor temperature during thermotherapy. Seven temperature sensors were taped to the skin and nipple to monitor the skin temperature during thermotherapy (see Figure 3.6). During treatment, the amount of breast compression, focused microwave power, and air cooling of the skin were adjusted to reduce or avoid pain for the patient—the microwave focusing is verified and adjusted as necessary after any change in breast compression. The maximum allowed thermotherapy treatment time was 60 minutes in this study. Patients were monitored for toxicity following treatment. Breast conservation surgery was to be performed within 60 days of thermotherapy.

8.2.3 Thermal Dose

Experimental studies support the concept that tumor cell heating for 60 minutes at 43°C is tumoricidal, and the period of time to kill tumor cells decreases by a factor of two for each degree increase in temperature above about 43°C.[3] During the tumor temperature increase above 43°C, thermal dose is accumulated in the tumor. The treatment time required for a 210-minute treatment at 43°C can be reduced, for example, to about 6.4 minutes at 48°C, 3.2 minutes at 49°C, or 1.6 minutes at 50°C, which is often referred to as equivalent thermal dose ($CEM_{43°C}$, cumulative equivalent minutes relative to 43°C). The cumulative equivalent minutes (CEM) thermal dose was calculated from the measured temperatures recorded by the sensor in the tumor and also for seven sensors on the skin and nipple—the desired tumor thermal dose during active microwave heating for this study was in the range of 140 to 180 $CEM_{43°C}$ at tumor temperatures in the range of 48° to 52°C.

To reach therapeutic temperature from the initial tumor temperature, the desired heating rate of the tumor was in the range of 1°C/minute to 2°C/minute. Once the desired temperature range and thermal dose range were achieved during active microwave heating (140 to 180 equivalent minutes), the microwave power was reduced to zero and breast compression was maintained during a 5-minute cooldown period. During the cooldown period, as a result of reduced blood flow from the breast compression and the thermal insulation of the surrounding breast tissues, the thermal dose continues to accumulate in the tumor toward the goal of a minimum of 210 thermal equivalent minutes.

8.2.4 Outcomes Measured

In this study, outcomes measured were pathologic margin status, surgical reexcision (intraoperative and second incision) rates, excised tissue volume, pathologic tumor necrosis, and focused microwave phased array (FMPA) thermotherapy–related side effects. Margins for the primary excision were assessed relative to multicolor inking to identify the medial, lateral, superior, inferior, anterior, and posterior aspects of the breast tissue. Tumor cell kill was based on tumor necrosis and was estimated from hematoxylin and eosin (H&E) histological sections (performed at each participating site) from wide local excision of the primary breast tumor. Necrosis was estimated and expressed as a percentage of necrotic tumor areas in relation to necrotic and viable tumor areas. If viable tumor cells were found either close (less than 1 mm from the inked margin) or at the inked margin, intraoperative reexcision was recommended by the pathologist.

Adverse events, vital signs, and laboratory measurements (complete blood count, blood urea nitrogen and creatinine, bilirubin, serum glutamic-oxaloacetic transaminase, serum glutamic-pyruvic transaminase, alkaline phosphatase, and routine chemistries) were monitored to evaluate the safety and tolerability of the thermal dose. Performance status was recorded after thermal therapy.

8.2.5 Statistical Analysis

Statistical differences between thermotherapy and surgery-alone groups were quantified using Student t test and Fisher's exact test (InStat, GraphPad Software, Inc.), as appropriate.[4] All tests were two-sided, and P values less than or equal to 0.05 were considered statistically significant. Parameters were quantified by mean, range, standard deviation (SD), and 95% confidence interval (CI) as appropriate. Cases excluded from statistical analysis included patients that did not receive treatment, patients with multifocal tumors, patients with extensive ductal carcinoma in situ (DCIS) determined by pathological evaluation of the excised breast tissue, patients discontinued or withdrawn from the study, patients that received an excisional biopsy, or patients with tumors not T1 or T2.

8.3 STUDY RESULTS

8.3.1 Patient Characteristics

A total of 92 patients were enrolled (46 in each arm), and 17 cases were excluded from statistical analysis, based on the criteria discussed in the previous section, providing a study group of 75 patients. In the thermotherapy arm, patients excluded from the study analysis were as follows: 1 patient had an excisional biopsy, 1 patient had a T3 tumor, 4 patients did not receive thermotherapy and withdrew from the study, 2 patients went on chemotherapy prior to surgery, 3 patients had multifocal tumors, and 1 patient had extensive DCIS. In the surgery alone arm, patients excluded were as follows: 1 patient signed informed consent but did not participate, 1 patient developed metastatic pancreatic cancer and was withdrawn from the study, and 3 patients had extensive DCIS. Demographics for the 75 patients included in the statistical analysis are summarized in **Table 8.1**. Thirty-four patients (mean age: 59.4, range 42–89 years) were treated with thermotherapy prior to surgery and 41 patients (mean age 58.0, range 41–89 years) received surgery alone ($P = 0.6$). At enrollment, mean tumor maximum diameter based on ultrasound was 1.7 cm (range 0.7 to 3.6 cm, 95% CI 1.5 to 1.9 cm) in the thermotherapy arm versus 1.6 cm (range 0.7 to 2.7 cm, 95% CI 1.4 to 1.8 cm) in the surgery-alone arm ($P = 0.49$). Clinically, in the thermotherapy arm there were 0% T1a (tumor greater than 0.1 cm but not greater than 0.5 cm), 20.6% T1b (tumor greater than 0.5 cm but not greater than 1.0 cm), 44.1% T1c (tumor greater than 1.0 cm but not greater than 2.0 cm), 35.3% T2 (tumor greater than 2.0 cm but not greater than 5.0 cm) tumors, and in the surgery-alone arm there were 2.4% T1a, 19.5% T1b, 53.7% T1c, 24.4% T2 tumors. Clinically, at enrollment in the thermotherapy arm 93.9% of patients were node negative and 6.1% were node positive, and in the surgery-alone arm 87.8% of patients were node negative and 12.2% were node positive. Based on pathologic final diagnosis, 32 of 34 (94%) patients in the thermotherapy arm had invasive ductal carcinomas compared with 37 of 41 (90%) patients in the surgery-alone arm ($P = 0.68$). DCIS was present in 12 of 34 (35.3%) patients in the thermotherapy arm compared to 25 of 41 (61%) in the surgery-alone arm ($P = 0.04$) at final diagnosis.

In the thermotherapy arm, 16 of 34 (47.0%) tumors were located laterally, 9 of 34 (26.5%) medially, and 9 of 34 (26.5%) at either the 6 o'clock or 12 o'clock position. In the surgery-alone arm, 19 of 41 (46.3%) tumors were located laterally, 12 of 41 (29.3%) medially, and 10 of 41 (24.4%) at either the 6 o'clock or 12 o'clock position.

In the thermotherapy arm, 79.4% of patients were postmenopausal compared to 73.2% in the surgery-alone arm. In the thermotherapy arm, 76.5% of patients were estrogen receptor (ER) positive, 50% progesterone receptor (PR) positive, and 21.2% HER-2/neu positive. In the surgery-alone arm, 82.8% of patients were ER positive, 75.6% were PR positive, and 34.1% were HER-2/neu positive.

Table 8.1 Demographic and Tumor Characteristics of the Study Population

		Thermotherapy	*Surgery Alone*
N		34	41
Age, Years	Mean	59.4	58.0
	Range	42–89	41–89
Tumor Size Based on Ultrasound Measurements at Enrollment	Mean, cm	1.7	1.6
	Range, cm	0.74–3.64	0.70–2.73
	95% Confidence Interval, cm	1.47–1.94	1.44–1.77
Clinical Tumor Classification at Enrollment	T1a	0%	2.4%
	T1b	20.6%	19.5%
	T1c	44.1%	53.7%
	T2	35.3%	24.4%
Clinical Nodal Status at Enrollment	Negative/Positive	93.9%/6.1%	87.8%/12.2%
Tumor Histology (final diagnosis)	Invasive ductal carcinoma	94%	90%
	Invasive lobular carcinoma	3%	7%
	Colloid	3%	3%
	DCIS component present	35%	61%
Tumor Grade (final diagnosis)	High Grade	40%	36%
	Intermediate Grade	43%	33%
	Low Grade	17%	31%

DCIS, ductal carcinoma in situ.

8.3.2 Thermotherapy Characteristics and Tumor Necrosis

The relevant thermal parameters and tumor necrosis results for the 34 thermotherapy-treated patients are summarized in **Table 8.2**. Breast compression at the start of thermotherapy had a mean value of 5.3 cm (range 3.0 to 9.2 cm, SD = 1.4 cm, 95% CI 4.8 to 5.9 cm). Microwave treatment time had a mean value of 26.6 minutes (range 5.0 to 60 minutes, SD = 14.9 minutes, 95% CI 21.4 to 31.8 minutes). The cumulative equivalent thermal dose had a mean value of 182.0 minutes (range 0 to 645.0 minutes, SD = 152.6 minutes, 95% CI 127.9 to 236.1 minutes). Microwave treatment energy dose (refer to Section 4.4) had a mean value of 150.7 kilojoules (range 28.8 to 350.3 kilojoules, SD = 88.5 kilojoules, 95% CI 139.3 to 192.1 kilojoules). Tumoricidal temperatures (> 43°C) were reached in 31 of 34 (91.2%) patients. The desired peak tumor temperature of (> 48°C) was achieved in 15 of 34 (44.1%) patients. The targeted thermal dose of 140 to 180 equivalent minutes during active microwave heating was achieved in 20 of 34 (58.8%) patients. With the additional tumor heating that occurred during the cooldown phase, the minimum desired thermal dose of 210 minutes was achieved in 17 of 34 (50%) patients. Patients underwent breast-conserving surgery on average 19.6 days after thermotherapy (range: 7–60 days, SD = 14.1 days, 95% CI 14.2 to 25.1 days). Twenty percent or more necrosis of breast cancer was achieved in 15 of 34 (44%) patients. Complete (100%) necrosis of invasive breast cancer was achieved in 2 of 34 (5.9%) cases. Mean pathologic tumor necrosis by volume was 29.8% (range 0% to 100%, SD = 38.7%, 95% CI 16.1 to 43.1%) in the thermotherapy arm and 0.1% (range 0% to 5%) in the surgery-alone arm ($P = 0.0001$).

In the group of 17 patients that received the minimum thermal dose of 210 equivalent minutes, the minimum targeted temperature of 48°C was achieved in 15 of 17 (88.2%) cases, and the mean tumor necrosis by volume for these 17 patients was 38.0% (range 0% to 100%). In this study, the most consistent high degree of tumor necrosis occurred when all of the following parameters occurred together: (1) a CEM thermal dose greater than 210 minutes was achieved in the tumor, (2) the tumor temperature was maintained above 48°C for greater than 2.0 minutes, (3) the microwave treatment time was

Table 8.2 Thermal Parameters and Tumor Necrosis Achieved in the Randomized Study

	Mean	Range	Standard Deviation	95% Confidence Interval
Breast Compression during Microwave Treatment (cm)	5.3	3.0–9.2	1.4	4.8–5.9
Microwave Treatment Time (minutes)	26.6	5.0–60.0	14.9	21.4–31.8
Microwave Energy Dose (kilojoules)	160.7	28.8–350.3	88.5	129.3–192.1
Peak Tumor Temperature (°C)	46.7	34.6–51.4	3.2	45.5–47.8
Time at Tumor Temperature >48°C (minutes)	1.2	0.0–5.2	1.66	0.6–1.8
Cumulative Thermal Dose CEM$_{43}$ (minutes)	182.0	0–645.0	152.6	127.9–236.1
Number of Days Between Thermotherapy and Surgery	19.6	7–60	14.1	14.2–25.1
% Tumor Necrosis (Thermotherapy)	29.8	0–100	38.7	16.1–43.1
% Tumor Necrosis (Control Arm)	0.1	0–5	0.8	0–0.4

CEM, cumulative equivalent minutes.

greater than 10 minutes, and (4) the microwave energy dose was greater than 50 kilojoules—five example cases meeting these parameters with tumor necrosis in the range of 90% to 100% are listed in **Table 8.3**. **Figure 8.1** shows an example of the measured tumor and surface temperatures versus time during treatment for Case 2421, in which the tumor temperature was elevated from a starting temperature of 33.3°C to a peak temperature of 48.7°C in 15.5 minutes. For this treatment, microwaves were turned off after 17.0 minutes when the thermal dose was 180 equivalent minutes and the tumor temperature was 48.2°C, and with 5-minute cooldown a cumulative thermal dose of 250.5 minutes was achieved at the end of treatment—the tumor ablation was 90% for this case. Measured surface temperatures were below 36°C throughout this treatment. For this case, the breast compression thickness at the start of thermotherapy treatment was 8.8 cm and the rate of tumor temperature increase was 0.8°C per minute during the first 5 minutes of treatment. Beginning at 5 minutes from the start of treatment, the breast compression was tightened to a thickness of 8.6 cm, which elevated the rate of tumor temperature increase to 1.3°C per minute. This case demonstrates that a small change in breast compression can significantly influence the rate of tumor heating—0.2-cm change in compression produced a 0.5°C per minute increase in the heating rate for the tumor.

Another case of note in Table 8.3 is Case 2608 in which microwaves were turned off when the thermal dose was 180 equivalent minutes at which time the peak temperature was 50.1°C. For this case, as the breast compression was maintained during the 5-minute cooldown, the tumor thermal dose continued to accumulate and the final cumulative thermal dose achieved was 529.7 equivalent minutes, that is, 349.7 thermal equivalent minutes were achieved during the cooldown period—100% tumor ablation was achieved for this case.

8.3.3 Excised Tissue and Margin Status

Predicted and actual excised breast tissue volumes and pathologic results for the thermotherapy arm and control arm are given in **Table 8.4**. At enrollment, based on ultrasound tumor measurements in three dimensions, the calculated mean tumor volume (Ellipsoidal volume = Length × Width × Depth × 0.524) was 2.5 cc in the ther-

Table 8.3 Thermotherapy Treatment Parameters, Tumor Necrosis, and Margin Status for Five Example Cases Listed by Increasing Tumor Necrosis

	Case 2421	Case 2511	Case 2609	Case 2802	Case 2608
Tumor Size (ultrasound at enrollment) (cm)	2.65	2.60	1.45	0.77	1.01
Breast Compression Thickness for Thermotherapy (cm)	8.8	4.0	5.0	7.0	6.5
Microwave Treatment Time (minutes)	17	11	21	24	13.5
Microwave Energy Dose (kilojoules)	122.6	70.0	109.8	156.0	59.4
Peak Tumor Temperature (°C)	48.7	48.4	48.6	48.1	50.1
Time at Tumor Temperature >48°C (minutes)	3.2	2.6	2.2	2.0	5.0
Cumulative Thermal Dose CEM_{43} (minutes) with Cooldown	250.5	230.7	220.2	240.0	529.7
Maximum Dimension of Tissue Excision (cm)	9.5	6.5	9.2	7.0	10.0
Tumor Necrosis by Volume	90%	98%	99%	100%	100%
Margin Status (negative, close, or positive)	Negative	Negative	Negative	Negative	Negative

CEM, cumulative equivalent minutes.

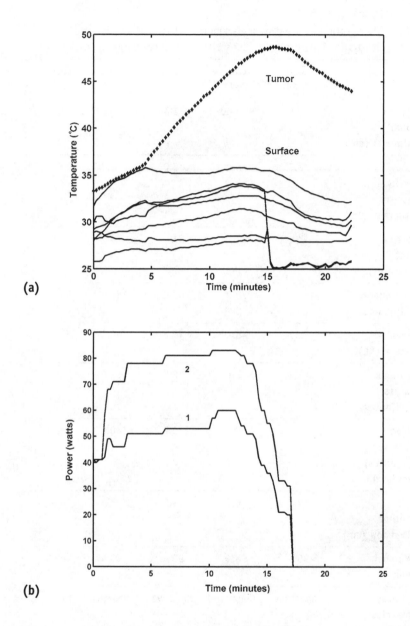

(a)

(b)

Figure 8.1   (a) Measured tumor and surface temperatures during thermotherapy treatment for Case 2421. (b) Commanded microwave power during treatment.

Table 8.4 Summary of Excised Tissue Volumes and Margin Status

		Thermo- therapy	Surgery Alone	
Number of Patients per Arm		34	41	P
Ultrasound-Measured Maximum Tumor Diameter at Enrollment (cm)	Mean	1.7	1.6	0.61
	Range	0.74–3.64	0.7–2.73	
	95% Confidence Interval	1.49–1.97	1.44–1.77	
Ultrasound-Measured Tumor Volume at Enrollment (cc)	Mean	2.5	1.5	0.14
	Range	0.13–14.12	0.1–6.7	
	95% Confidence Interval	1.33–3.58	1.05–2.03	
Predicted Breast Tissue Excision Volume Based on 2-cm Margin Surrounding Elliptical Tumor Measured by Ultrasound in Three Dimensions (cc)	Mean	88.7	80.4	0.18
	Range	52.4–182.6	50.2–133.8	
	95% Confidence Interval	77.9–99.5	73.9–86.8	
Number of Inter- operative Reexcisions per Patient	Mean	0.74	0.71	0.88
Margin Status at Completion of First Surgery	Rate of negative margins	29/34 (85.3%)	30/41 (73.2%)	0.26
	Rate of close margins	5/34 (14.7%)	7/41 (17.1%)	0.81
	Rate of positive margins	0/34 (0%)	4 of 41 (9.8%)	0.13
	Rate of close or positive margins	5/34 (14.7%)	11/41 (26.8%)	0.26
Incidence Rate for Type of Tumor Cells Involved in Close or Positive Final Margins (invasive only, DCIS only, or both invasive and DCIS) for First Surgery	Invasive only	3/34 (8.8%)	7/41 (17.1%)	0.33
	DCIS only	0/34 (0%)	4/41 (9.8%)	0.13
	Both invasive and DCIS	2/34 (5.9%)	0/41 (0%)	0.20
Rate of Second Incisions		2/34 (5.9%)	4/41 (9.8%)	0.68
Pathology-Measured Maximum Tumor Diameter from Excised Specimen (cm)	Mean	1.87	1.85	0.94
	Range	0.0–4.5	0.8–3.3	
	95% Confidence Interval	1.5–2.2	1.6–2.1	

(continues)

Table 8.4 Summary of Excised Tissue Volumes and Margin Status (continued)

Pathology-Measured Maximum Tissue Diameter of Excised Specimen (cm)	Mean	8.3	7.4	0.07
	Range	4.5–14.0	3.0–11.7	
	95% Confidence Interval	7.6–9.0	6.7–8.1	
Pathology-Measured Tumor Volume from Excised Specimen (cc)	Mean	3.24	3.05	0.82
	Range	0–13.95	0.15–14.15	
	95% Confidence Interval	2.0–4.47	1.98–4.12	
Actual Breast Tissue Excision Volume Including First Excision and All Reexcisions (cc)	Mean	117.8	94.7	0.13
	Range	24.3–363.1	4.4–282.0	
	95% Confidence Interval	93.7–141.9	75.1–114.2	
% Excess Breast Tissue (by volume) Excised Compared to Predicted	Mean	41.7	16.5	0.18
	Range	−65 to 253	−94 to 240.9	
	95% Confidence Interval	12.0 to 71.5	−6.5 to 39.4	

DCIS = ductal carcinoma in situ.
$P > .05$ not significant.

motherapy arm and 1.5 cc in the surgery-alone arm ($P = 0.14$). Assuming a 2-cm surgical margin surrounding the ellipsoidal tumor, the predicted mean volume of excised breast tissue was 88.7 cc in the thermotherapy arm and 80.4 cc in the surgery-alone arm ($P = 0.18$). The mean ellipsoidal volume of excised breast tissue in the first surgery, including any intraoperative reexcisions, was 115.0 cc (range 24.3 to 363.1 cc, 95% CI 91.2 to 139.0 cc) in the thermotherapy arm and 90.7 cc (range 4.4 to 282.0 cc, 95% CI 71.4 to 110.0 cc) in the surgery-alone arm ($P = 0.11$). The rate of intraoperative reexcisions during the first surgery was 0.74 per patient in the thermotherapy arm and 0.71 per patient in the surgery-alone arm ($P = 0.88$).

Based on gross pathology, the maximum dimension of excised breast tumor had a mean value of 1.87 cm (range 0 to 4.5 cm, 95% CI 1.5 to 2.2 cm) in the thermotherapy arm and 1.85 cm (range 0.8 to 3.3 cm, 95% CI 1.6 to 2.1 cm) in the surgery-alone arm ($P = 0.94$). The gross maximum dimension of the initial excised breast tissue (prior to any reexcisions) had a mean value of 8.3 cm (range 4.5 to 14.0 cm, 95% CI 7.6 to 9.0 cm) in the thermotherapy arm and 7.4 cm (range 3.0 to 11.7 cm, 95% CI 6.7 to 8.1 cm) in the surgery-alone arm ($P = 0.07$, close to statistical significance).

The mean volume of excised breast carcinoma from gross pathology in the first surgery was 3.2 cc (range 0.0 to 13.9 cc, 95% CI 2.0 to 4.4 cc) in the thermotherapy arm and 3.1 cc (range 0.2 to 4.1 cc, 95% CI 2.0 to 4.1 cc) in the surgery-alone arm ($P = 0.9$). The mean volume of excised breast tissue, including first excision and all reexcisions, was 117.8 cc (range 24.3 to 363.1 cc, 95% CI 93.7 to 141.9 cc) in the thermotherapy arm and 94.7 cc (range 4.4 to 282.0 cc, 95% CI 75.1 to 114.2%) in the surgery-alone arm ($P = 0.13$).

In the thermotherapy arm, 5 of 34 (14.7%) patients had close or positive margins (five were close, none were positive), whereas in the surgery-alone arm 11 of 41 (26.8%) patients had close or positive margins (seven were close, four were positive) ($P = 0.26$). In the thermotherapy arm, 5 of 34 (14.7%) patients had close margins, and in the surgery-alone arm 7 of 41 (17.1%) had close margins ($P = 0.81$). In the thermotherapy arm, 0 of 34 (0%) patients had positive margins, and in the surgery-alone arm 4 of 41 (9.8%) patients had positive margins ($P = 0.13$). Of the five patients with close margins in the thermotherapy arm, three cases involved invasive ductal carcinoma cells close to the margins, and two cases had both invasive and intraductal carcinomas close to the margins. Of the 11 patients in the surgery-alone arm with close or positive margins, 7 cases involved only invasive carcinoma at the margins and 4 cases involved only DCIS at the margins. In the thermotherapy arm, 2 of 34 (5.9%) patients received a second incision, and in the surgery-alone arm 4 of 41 (9.8%) patients received a second incision ($P = 0.68$).

8.3.4 Side Effects

In this study, 3 of 34 (8.5%) patients receiving thermotherapy had a skin burn less than 3 cm in size that, in each case, was excised during the subsequent breast-conserving surgery procedure. These three patients received peak skin temperatures of 44.2°C, 42.4°C, 41.7°C and skin thermal doses of 5.7, 1.5, 2.7 minutes, respectively. During thermotherapy treatment, 22 of 34 (64.7%) patients had no pain, 3 of 34 (8.8%) had mild pain, 7 of 34 (20.6%) had moderate pain, and 2 of 34 (5.9%) had severe pain. With respect to the overall thermotherapy treatment, 15 of 34 (44.1%) patients had no discomfort during thermotherapy, 11 of 34 (32.4%) had mild discomfort, 3 of 34 (8.8%) had moderate discomfort, and 5 of 34 (14.7%) had intolerable discomfort. During thermotherapy treatment, 3 of 34 (8.8%) patients experienced nausea. None of the patients (0 of 34 [0%]) in the thermotherapy arm developed a fever, hypotension, dizziness, or ulceration as a result of thermotherapy. Skin reddening (erythema) occurred in 4 of 34 (11.8%) patients as a result of the mechanical compression of the skin or from microwave treatment. Edema was reported in 3 of 34 (8.8%) cases. Moderate skin ecchymosis possibly related to thermotherapy occurred in 1 of 34 (2.9%) patients—the event resolved within 9 days. Mild nipple retraction possibly related to thermotherapy occurred in 1 of 34 (2.9%) patients. Mild subcutaneous fibrosis occurred in 1 of 34 (2.9%) patients. Moderate abscess caused by necrotic tissue surrounding the tumor occurred in 1 of 34 (2.9%) patients—the patient was given antibiotics and the wound was irrigated, and the event was resolved within 29 days. Hematoma/seroma was reported in 6 of 34 (17.6%) thermotherapy patients—3 cases were mild, 2 cases were mild/moderate, and 1 case was moderate severity.

Incomplete thermotherapy treatments, in which the thermal dose did not reach 140 to 180 minutes during microwave heating, occurred because of pain or discomfort in 10 of 34 (29.4%) patients—intolerable discomfort (5 cases with tumor thermal doses of 5.25, 12.6, 30.9, 55.0, and 90.1 minutes), moderate pain (1 case with tumor thermal dose 23.7 minutes), and mild pain (4 cases with tumor thermal doses of 6.6, 50.9, 68.3, and 81.5 minutes). Four (4) other cases with incomplete thermotherapy treatments were skin temperature rising too quickly (1 case with tumor thermal dose of 18.0 minutes, no pain or discomfort), temperature sensor not in tumor (1 case with tumor thermal dose not measured, no pain or discomfort), patient with a small breast and the tumor could not be heated (1 case with tumor thermal dose of 0 minutes, no pain or discomfort), tumor close to nipple and nipple heating too rapidly (1 case with tumor thermal dose of 3.5 minutes, no pain or discomfort). Three (3) cases with thermal doses of 178.5, 198.0, and 207.6 equivalent minutes (with corresponding peak tumor temperatures 46.3°C, 47.4°C, and 47.9°C) did not reach the desired 210-minute dose or the minimum peak tumor temperature 48°C and were associated with mild discomfort from the thermotherapy procedure.

8.4 DISCUSSION

There is an increasing interest in the use of minimally invasive ablative techniques in the treatment of breast cancer.[5] A new treatment paradigm in which systemic therapy may be followed by minimally invasive local therapy to eradicate any residual local tumor has been proposed and is the subject of research studies. This paradigm is seen as the next step in an evolution of therapy that is designed to offer less-invasive means of therapy to patients presenting with small cancers that are detected as a result of screening practices.

The objective of using minimally invasive treatment techniques is to cause complete local tumor regression and long-term local control of breast cancer with minimal damage to the surrounding normal breast tissue and the skin. Other characteristics of the ideal treatment are that it must be an outpatient procedure using a percutaneous or transcutaneous application without the need of sedation or general anesthesia. The morbidity and local complications must be minimal. Thermal ablation has taken a prominent role in minimally invasive approaches to treat neoplasms.[5] Heat energy can be generated by the use of radiofrequency,[6] interstitial laser photocoagulation,[7] focused ultrasound,[8] and focused microwaves[2] for elevated temperature tumor ablation, whereas freezing can be achieved through cryoablation.[9] The cytotoxic effects of thermotherapy on cancer cells using temperatures in the range of at least 45° to 53°C have been demonstrated on cancer cells in vitro.[10]

In this clinical trial of preoperative thermotherapy, 15 of 34 (44%) thermotherapy patients exhibited various degrees of coagulative tumor necrosis that ranged from 20% to 100%. Based on H&E staining, complete (100%) necrosis of breast cancer was achieved in 2 of 34 (5.9%) cases—in both of these cases there was no evidence of viable invasive carcinoma or DCIS cells. Tumor cell kill measured by other pathologic testing such as nicotinamide adenine dinucleotide-diaphorase and immunohistochemistry, as used in other breast tumor ablation studies,[11,12] were not evaluated in this study. The main objective of this study of FMPA thermotherapy was to determine whether a cumulative thermal dose of 210 minutes or more could cause tumor ablation and a decrease in the rate of positive margins without clinically significant toxicity in a multicenter randomized setting. The target cumulative thermal dose of 210 equivalent minutes was achieved in 17 of 34 (50%) patients, and the desired peak tumor temperature of greater than 48°C was achieved in 15 of 34 (44.1%) patients. A reduction in the incidence of positive margins was suggested in the thermotherapy arm; however, both consistent delivery of the targeted tumor thermal dose and consistent tumor necrosis were not achieved in this study. A lack of consistency in achieving the desired thermal dose was because of pain in 29.4% of cases and because of other factors in the remaining 21.6% of cases—some of the cases in which the desired thermal treatment was not achieved might be a result of the learning curve associated with using a new treatment technology in a multi-institutional study.

An observation arising from this study is the 0% rate of positive margins in the thermotherapy arm in comparison to 9.8% positive margins in the surgery-alone arm and reported incidences of positive margins after breast-conserving surgery in the literature of 4% to 44%.[13-16] However, this difference in positive margins did not reach statistical significance and might be the result of a type 2 statistical error requiring a larger clinical trial to demonstrate a statistical difference. Therefore, the hypothesis that FMPA thermotherapy treatment prior to breast conservation surgery provides significant tumor cell kill in the primary tumor and in the margins and is responsible for a low incidence of positive margins requires further critical study. Two other factors might be responsible for this finding regarding positive margins:

1. A smaller volume of breast tissue on average was excised in the surgery-alone arm and might have contributed to a higher rate of positive margins in the surgery-alone arm compared to pre-operative thermotherapy. Possible explanations for the larger volume of breast tissue excised in the thermotherapy arm might include increased firmness (induration) of the breast cancer mass as a result of thermotherapy effects leading to better resection, or investigator bias because this was not a blinded study. Future studies of focused microwave thermotherapy could investigate whether induration of the breast tumor occurs more frequently in the thermotherapy arm compared to surgery alone.

2. At final pathologic diagnosis, a higher rate of DCIS (61% in the surgery-alone arm versus 35.3% in the thermotherapy arm [$P = 0.04$], based on pathology) might have been a contributing factor to the higher rate of positive margins in the surgery-alone arm compared to thermotherapy. Elements of intraductal carcinoma might extend outside the tumor mass and can be difficult to detect preoperatively with mammography.[17] This characteristic of DCIS is a potential pitfall of minimally invasive ablative approaches. In addition, microwave-heating properties of DCIS lesions need to be evaluated in future studies to determine whether DCIS is high-water-, high-ion-content similar to invasive breast carcinomas. Studies demonstrate that the differentiation of DCIS is correlated with the grade of the associated invasive ductal carcinoma,[18,19] indicating a pathological similarity between DCIS and invasive ductal carcinoma cells. If microwave thermotherapy does not preferentially heat DCIS, then DCIS might be a potential exclusion criterion. Future studies of thermal ablation must consider selecting patients with invasive carcinoma with lower risk of an intraductal carcinoma component based on pretreatment mammography and percutaneous biopsy results.[19,20] Future studies could determine whether FMPA thermotherapy has an ablative effect on DCIS.

The ability of FMPA thermotherapy to consistently deliver a specified therapeutic thermal dose and minimum temperature to breast tumors and achieve consistent 100% pathologic tumor cell kill might depend on a number of factors, including (1) breast compression thickness, which impacts blood flow in the tumor and in surrounding tissues, and the required penetration depth for the microwaves, (2) tumor size, (3) tumor histology, (4) tumor location, (5) accuracy, number and positioning of tumor temperature probes, (6) initial temperature of tumor, (7) magnitude of surface cooling, (8) patient pain tolerance, (9) length of time between thermotherapy and surgery, and (10) method of pathologic evaluation of tumor cell kill.

It would be desirable in future clinical studies of focused microwave breast thermotherapy to explore a more consistent delivery of a minimum 210-minute thermal dose (with a corresponding peak tumor temperature in the range of about 48° to 50°C) and higher thermal doses for more effective tumor cell kill based on necrosis. Future studies of FMPA thermotherapy could explore measuring the tumor blood perfusion rate with Doppler ultrasound when the breast is compressed prior to the start of thermotherapy to assess the ability to overcome perfusion effects and more effectively heat the tumor— these perfusion measurements could be used as a guide to determine the desired breast compression thickness prior to the start of thermotherapy. Future studies conducted at more consistent and/or higher therapeutic doses of FMPA will provide meaningful information regarding the success of this therapy for heat-alone treatment of breast cancer based on pathological response. Comparison with other means of percutaneous thermal ablation of breast cancer will then be possible.

Approaches to measure the success of thermal ablation are essential if a nonsurgical management is contemplated. Imaging with mammography is unlikely to provide additional valuable information. Ultrasound is most valuable in providing easy targeting and placement of the sensors within the mass, but might not provide information about the viability of the tumor. On the other hand, delayed contrast-enhanced magnetic resonance imaging has the potential to show the effects of treatment as areas of devascularization (nonenhancement) within the treated area.[21] Alternatively, more extensive tissue sampling in follow-up with core biopsy or vacuum-assisted core biopsy can provide essential information of residual tumor.

In the current study, FMPA was conducted by the placement of a percutaneous sensor catheter for focusing of the microwaves (E-field sensor) and measurement of tumor temperatures (temperature sensor). In the future, FMPA has the potential of being a transcutaneous procedure that does not require the insertion of any needle-type devices, and targeting might be conducted based on imaging alone.

In the present study,[1] thermal ablation with FMPA was well tolerated and no significant complications were recorded.

8.5 SUMMARY

This chapter described a randomized clinical trial in which patients received either preoperative focused microwave thermotherapy prior to breast-conserving surgery in the new arm or breast-conserving surgery alone in the control arm. The results were suggestive of an improvement in margin status and second incision rate in the preoperative thermotherapy plus breast-conserving surgery arm, but a larger study is required to verify this conclusion.

REFERENCES

1. Dooley WC, Vargas HI, Fenn, AJ, et al. Randomized study of preoperative focused microwave phased array thermotherapy for early-stage invasive breast cancer. To be submitted to *Ann Surg Oncol.*

2. Vargas HI, Dooley WC, Gardner RA, Gonzalez KD, Venegas R, Heywang-Kobrunner SH, Fenn AJ. Focused microwave phased array thermotherapy for ablation of early-stage breast cancer: results of thermal dose escalation. *Ann Surg Oncol.* 2004;11(2):139–146.

3. Sapareto SA, Dewey WC. Thermal dose determination in cancer therapy. *Int J Radiat Oncol Biol Phys.* 1984;10:787–800.

4. Armitage P, Berry G. *Statistical Methods in Medical Research.* 3rd ed. Oxford, England: Blackwell Science; 1994:156–163, 283–311.

5. Singletary SE. Minimally invasive techniques in breast cancer treatment. *Seminars in Surg Onc.* 2001;20:246–250.

6. Izzo F, Thomas R, Delrio P, *et al.* Radiofrequency ablation in patients with primary breast carcinoma. A pilot study of 26 patients. *Cancer.* 2001;92:2036–2044.

7. Dowlatshashi K, Francescatti DS, Bloom KJ. Laser therapy for small breast cancers. *Am J Surg.* 2002;184:359–363.

8. Huber PE, Jenne JW, Rastert R, et al. A new noninvasive approach in breast cancer therapy using magnetic resonance imaging–guided focused ultrasound surgery. *Cancer Res.* 2001;61:8441–8447.

9. Pfleiderer SO, Freesmeyer MG, Marx C, Kuhne-Heid R, Schneider A, Kaiser WA. Cryotherapy of breast cancer under ultrasound guidance: initial results and limitations. *Eur Radiol.* 2002;12:3009–3014.

10. Gerhard H, Klinger HG, Gabriel E. Short term hyperthermia: in vitro survival of different human cell lines after short exposure to extreme temperatures. In: Streffer C, Beuningen D, Dietzel F, et al, eds. *Cancer Therapy by Hyperthermia and Radiation.* Baltimore, Md: Urban & Schwarzenberg; 1978:201–203.

11. Gardner RA, Vargas HI, Block JB, Vogel CL, Fenn AJ, Kuehl GV, Doval M. Focused microwave phased array thermotherapy for primary breast cancer. *Ann Surg Oncol.* 2002;9(4):326–332.

12. Huston TL, Simmons RM. Ablative therapies for the treatment of malignant diseases of the breast. *Am J Surg.* 2005;189:694–701.

13. Recht A, Come SE, Henderson IC, et al. The sequencing of chemotherapy and radiation therapy after conservative surgery for early stage breast cancer. *N Engl J Med.* 1996;334:1356–1361.

14. Park CC, Mitsumori M, Nixon A, et al. Outcome at 8 years after breast-conserving surgery and radiation therapy for invasive breast cancer: influence of margin status and systemic therapy on local recurrence. *J Clin Oncol.* 2000;18: 1668–1675.

15. Smitt MC, Nowels KW, Zdeblick MJ. The importance of lumpectomy surgical margin status in long term results of breast conservation. *Cancer.* 1995;76: 259–267.

16. Ryoo MC, Kagan AT, Wollin M, et al. Prognostic factors for recurrence and cosmesis in 393 patients after radiation therapy for early mammary carcinoma. *Radiology.* 1989;172:555–559.

17. Holland R, Hendriks JH, Vebeek AL, Mravunac M, Schuurmans Stekhoven JH. Extent, distribution, and mammographic/histological correlations of breast ductal carcinoma in situ. *Lancet.* 1990;335:519–522.

18. Douglas-Jones AG, Gupta SK, Attanoos RL, Morgan JM, Mansel RE. A critical appraisal of six modern classifications of ductal carcinoma in situ of the breast (DCIS): correlation with grade of associated invasive carcinoma. *Histopathology.* 1996;29:397–409.

19. Cadman B, Ostrowski J, Quinn C. Invasive ductal carcinoma accompanied by ductal carcinoma *in situ* (DCIS): comparison of DCIS grade with grade of invasive component. *The Breast.* 1997;6:132–137.

20. Bagnall MJ, Evans AJ, Wilson AR, et al. Predicting invasion in mammographically detected microcalcification. *Clin Radiol.* 2001;56:828–832.

21. Hall-Craggs MA. Interventional MRI of the breast: minimally invasive therapy. *Eur Radiol.* 2000;10:59–62.

Randomized Study of Preoperative Focused Microwave Thermotherapy in Combination with Preoperative Anthracycline-Based Chemotherapy for Patients with Large Breast Carcinomas

CHAPTER

9

9.1 INTRODUCTION

In Section 1.5 in Chapter 1, for patients with large breast cancer tumors, a clinical rationale for the combination of focused microwave thermotherapy and neoadjuvant chemotherapy was given. The clinical rationale is based on large randomized clinical studies of preoperative chemotherapy[1-4] for patients with operable breast cancer that show improved tumor response, and that thermotherapy is synergistic with chemotherapy with an intent for higher tumor response when the two modalities are combined. A randomized clinical study[5] was undertaken to determine whether focused microwave thermotherapy could be safely administered in combination with neoadjuvant anthracycline (AC)–based chemotherapy in patients with large breast carcinomas and whether an improvement in tumor response could be measured.

165

9.2 PATIENTS, MATERIALS, AND METHODS

Between November 2002 and May 2004, patients with primary invasive T2 (2- to 5-cm clinical diameter), or T3 (> 5-cm clinical diameter) breast carcinomas seen at (1) University of Oklahoma, Oklahoma City; (2) Harbor-UCLA Medical Center, Torrance, California; (3) Comprehensive Breast Center, Coral Springs, Florida; (4) Mroz-Baier Breast Care Center, Memphis, Tennessee; (5) Pearl Place, Tacoma, Washington; (6) St. Joseph's Hospital, Orange, California; (7) Breast Care Specialists, Norfolk, Virginia; (8) Breast Care, Las Vegas, Nevada; and (9) Carolina Surgery, Gastonia, North Carolina, were invited to participate in this Food and Drug Administration (FDA)–approved clinical study of the use of focused microwaves in combination with neoadjuvant AC-based chemotherapy compared with neoadjuvant AC-based chemotherapy alone. This study was approved and monitored by the Human Subjects Committee at each participating institution. Eligibility criteria included (1) Karnofski performance status > 70%, (2) core-needle-biopsy-proven invasive breast cancer, (3) patient was a candidate for mastectomy and was eligible for neoadjuvant chemotherapy treatment, (4) visible tumor measurable by clinical exam and by ultrasound, and (5) absence of involvement of the skin or pectoralis muscle. All patients were required to undergo counseling and to sign written informed consent forms.

Specific exclusion criteria were pregnancy, breast-feeding, and presence of breast implants, pacemakers or defibrillators. Other exclusion criteria were (1) known bleeding diathesis, (2) laboratory evidence of coagulopathy (prothrombin, international normalized ratio > 1.5; partial prothrombin > 1.5), (3) thrombocytopenia (platelet count < 100,000/mm^3), (4) anticoagulant therapy, or (5) evidence of chronic liver disease or renal failure.

Patients randomized to thermotherapy were scheduled to receive four cycles (every 21 days) of standard AC chemotherapy (doxorubicin at 60 mg/m^2 and cyclophosphamide at 600 mg/m^2) and two cycles of focused microwave thermotherapy typically on the same day as the first two cycles of AC chemotherapy—thermotherapy was to be administered typically starting within 1 to 4 hours after chemotherapy was infused, but no later than 36 hours after chemotherapy. Microwave treatment was performed on an outpatient basis using local anesthesia with patients in the prone position. An FDA-approved two-channel 915-MHz (megahertz) focused microwave adaptive phased array thermotherapy system (Microfocus-1000 APA; Celsion [Canada] Limited, Ontario, Canada) was used in this study (see Figure 3.4).[6] This minimally invasive treatment system produces a wide-focused microwave field in the compressed breast to heat and destroy high-water-content tumor tissue and tumor cells in the margins up to about 8 to 10 cm in maximum dimension. A 16-gauge (1.65-mm OD, 1.22-mm ID) closed-end plastic catheter was inserted into the tumor under ultrasound guidance, and a single-use disposable combination E-field focusing sensor and temperature sensor (1.12-mm OD) was inserted in the catheter to focus the microwaves and measure the tumor temperature during thermotherapy (see Figure 3.5). Seven temperature sensors were taped to the skin and nipple to monitor the surface temperature during thermotherapy (see Figure 3.6). During thermotherapy treatment, the amount of breast compression, focused microwave power, and air cooling of the skin were adjusted to reduce or avoid pain for the patient—the microwave focusing is verified and adjusted as necessary after any change in breast compression. The maximum allowed thermotherapy treatment time was 60 minutes in this study. Patients were monitored for toxicity following treatment.

Experimental studies support the concept that tumor cell heating for 60 minutes at 43°C is tumoricidal, and the period of time to kill tumor cells decreases by a factor of two for each degree increase in temperature above about 43°C.[7] During the tumor temperature increase above 43°C, thermal dose is accumulated in the tumor. The actual treatment time required for a 100-minute treatment at 43°C can be reduced, for example, to about 50 minutes at 44°C, 25 minutes at 44°C, or 12.5 minutes at 46°C, which is often referred to as equivalent thermal dose (CEM$_{43°C}$, cumulative equivalent minutes relative to 43°C). The cumulative equivalent minutes (CEM) thermal dose was calculated from the measured temperatures recorded by the sensor in the tumor—the desired tumor thermal dose during active microwave heating for this study was in the range of 80 to 120 CEM$_{43°C}$ in each of two treatments, at tumor temperatures in the range of 44° to 46°C. To reach therapeutic temperature from the initial tumor temperature, the desired heating rate of the tumor is in the range of 1° to 2°C/minute. Once the desired temperature range and thermal dose range is achieved during active microwave heating, the microwave power is reduced to zero and breast compression is maintained during a 5-minute cooldown period. During the cooldown period, as a result of reduced blood flow from the breast compression and the thermal insulation of the surrounding breast tissues, the thermal dose continues to accumulate in the tumor while the surface temperatures quickly resume normal values. Based on two such thermotherapy treatments, the desired cumulative thermal dose would have a range of 160 to 240 $CEM_{43°C}$ and should provide a significant tumor response because a heat-alone thermal dose of 210 minutes or greater (relative to 43°C) is predictive of 100% necrosis for invasive breast carcinomas.[6]

Breast tumor response was quantified by clinical exam in two dimensions (area = product of two diameters) and by ultrasound measurements in three dimensions (elliptical volume = length × width × depth × 0.524). Tumor cell kill was based on tumor necrosis and was estimated from hematoxylin and eosin (H&E) histological sections (performed at each participating site) from the excised breast tumor. Necrosis was estimated and expressed as a percentage of necrotic tumor areas in relation to necrotic and viable tumor areas.

9.3 RESULTS

A total of 34 adult female patients with T2, T3 invasive breast cancer were enrolled in this study. Seventeen (17) patients were randomized to the thermochemotherapy group and 17 were randomized to the chemotherapy-alone group. As a result of changes in standard-of-care neoadjuvant chemotherapy that occurred at some of the sites during this trial, the trial was closed early; however, key findings are discussed here.

9.3.1 Comparison of Thermochemotherapy Arm and Chemotherapy-Alone Arm for the Overall Study Population

Accounting for two patients that were withdrawn from the thermochemotherapy arm, data for 15 of 17 patients in that arm could be analyzed. In the chemotherapy-alone arm, 4 patients were withdrawn, leaving 13 cases for analysis.

As listed in **Table 9.1**, 15 patients (mean age 45.1 years, range 26 to 72 years, 6 T2 and 9 T3 tumors) received thermotherapy and AC chemotherapy prior to surgery, and 13 patients (mean age 45.8 years, range 32 to 69 years, 9 T2 and 4 T3 tumors) received AC chemotherapy alone prior to surgery. In the thermochemotherapy arm at enrollment, mean breast tumor diameter was 5.26 cm (range 2.4 to 7.5 cm) based on clinical examination and was 3.65 cm (range 2.0 to 7.8 cm) with volume 22.09 cc (range 1.85 to 90.98 cc) based on ultrasound measurements. In the chemotherapy-alone arm at enrollment, mean breast tumor diameter was 4.19 cm (range 2.5 to 9 cm) based on clinical examination and was 2.69 cm (range 1.22 to 6.5 cm) with volume 10.37 cc (range 0.39 to 78.68 cc) based on ultrasound measurements. At enrollment the difference in the median clinical tumor size in the two arms was statistically significant ($P = 0.05$), as was the difference in ultrasound tumor volume ($P = 0.02$).

In the thermochemotherapy arm, the mean peak tumor temperature achieved was 45.0°C (range 44.6° to 46.5°C), and the mean tumor thermal dose was 147.8 minutes (range 0 to 233.9 minutes). Objective tumor response in terms of median percentage of tumor shrinkage based on ultrasound measurements is summarized in **Table 9.2**. In the thermochemotherapy arm prior to surgery, the mean tumor diameter was 1.53 cm (range 0 to 3.5 cm) and volume was 3.13 cc (range 0 to 16.43 cc) based on ultrasound—mean tumor shrinkage compared to the volume at enrollment was 69.6% with median value 88.4% ($n = 14$) based on ultrasound-measured volume. In the chemotherapy-alone arm prior to surgery, the mean tumor diameter based on ultrasound was 1.97 cm (range 1.0 to 4.54 cm) and volume was 4.36 cc (range 0.24 to 13.28 cc) based on ultrasound—mean tumor shrinkage was 50.5% with median value 58.8% ($n = 10$) based on ultrasound-measured volume. In this study, there was a statistically significant increase in the median value of absolute tumor shrinkage (88.4% vs. 58.8%, $P = 0.048$, Mann-Whitney two-sided test) for preoperative thermochemotherapy compared to preoperative chemotherapy alone. As a result of the thermochemotherapy treatments, 14 of 15 (93.3%) patients had sufficient tumor shrinkage in the breast to become eligible (in principle) for breast conservation and 11 of 15 (73.3%) patients actually received breast conservation surgery. In the chemotherapy-alone arm, 12 of 13 (92.3%) patients were eligible and actually received breast conservation surgery. Comparing the actual breast conservation rates (11 of 15 in the thermochemotherapy arm versus 12 of 13

Table 9.1 Demographic and Tumor Characteristics of the Overall Study Population

		Thermochemo-therapy	Chemotherapy Alone
N		15	13
Age (years)	Mean	45.1	45.8
	Range	26–72	32–79
Menopausal Status	Pre	11	9
	Post	4	4
Tumor Size Based on Ultrasound Measurements at Enrollment	Mean, cm	3.65	2.69
	Range, cm	2.0–7.8	1.22 to 6.5
Tumor Size Based on Clinical Measurements at Enrollment	Mean, cm	5.26	4.19
	Range, cm	2.4–7.5	2.5–9.0
Clinical Tumor Classification at Enrollment	T2	6	9
	T3	9	4
Clinical Nodal Status at Enrollment	Negative	10	7
	Positive	5	6
Tumor Histology	Invasive ductal carcinoma	11	12
	Invasive lobular carcinoma	3	0
	Invasive, mixed ductal/lobular	1	1
Hormonal Receptor Status	ER negative	8	4
	ER positive	7	9
	PR negative	10	8
	PR positive	5	5
HER-2 Status	Negative	8	11
	Positive	6	2
	Unknown	1	0

HER-2 (human epidermal growth factor receptor 2)

Table 9.2 Median Tumor Shrinkage for Chemotherapy-Alone (Control) Arm and Thermochemotherapy Arm of the Overall Study Population

Study Parameter	Preoperative Chemotherapy (Control Arm n = 10)	Preoperative Thermochemotherapy (New Arm n = 14)	P value
Tumor shrinkage based on ultrasound volume (median)	58.8%	88.4%	0.048

in the chemotherapy-alone arm) statistically using Fisher's exact test, the two-sided *P* value is 0.33 (not significant). Of the patients receiving thermochemotherapy, mean pathologic tumor necrosis by volume was 72.6% (range 0% to 100%, $n = 14$) with two patients having a complete pathologic response, and in the chemotherapy-alone arm mean pathologic tumor necrosis by volume was 45.7% (range 0% to 100%, $n = 7$), $P = 0.41$.

For all T2, T3 tumors in this study, side effects caused by thermotherapy were as follows: fever did not occur for any subjects. Erythema (temporary skin redness) occurred in 6 of 26 (23.1%) treatments. A skin burn (less than 1.5 cm in size) in the microwave treatment field occurred in 5 of 26 (19.2%) treatments (Cases 1102, 1403, 1406, 1410, and 1703)—in each case, the peak skin temperature exceeded 40°C (range 40.4° to 42.5°C). The subject's level of discomfort with thermotherapy reported for 22 treatments was 5 of 22 (22.7%) no discomfort, 11 of 22 (50.0%) mild discomfort, 5 of 22 (22.7%) moderate discomfort, and 1 of 22 (4.5%) intolerable discomfort.

Based on the preceding comparison, preoperative thermotherapy can be administered safely in combination with four cycles of preoperative AC chemotherapy for patients with T2, T3 breast carcinomas with minimal morbidity. Thermochemotherapy had a greater tumor response in terms of shrinkage compared to chemotherapy alone for T2, T3 tumors. However, it was observed that the actual rate of breast conservation was very high in the chemotherapy arm and the tumors at enrollment were smaller than in the thermochemotherapy arm (with statistical significance). It can be hypothesized that larger tumors, 3.5 cm or larger based on clinical exam, might have an improved response rate in terms of shrinkage and tumor necrosis with preoperative thermochemotherapy treatment compared to preoperative chemotherapy-alone treatment. A subset of the preceding thermochemotherapy patient database, for tumors 3.5 cm and larger based on clinical exam, is analyzed from a safety standpoint in the next section.

9.3.2 Thermochemotherapy in Subset Group of Tumors, 3.5 cm or Larger

Demographics for a subset of thermochemotherapy-treated patients with clinical tumors 3.5 cm or larger analyzed in this study are summarized in **Table 9.3**. Seven patients (mean age 45.2, range 26–62 years) with T2, T3 invasive breast carcinomas received two thermotherapy treatments in combination with the first two of four planned AC chemotherapy treatments. Two patients were clinically node positive, and five were node negative. Six patients were estrogen receptor (ER) negative, and six patients were progesterone receptor (PR) negative—the remaining patient was both ER and PR positive. One patient (14.3%) was HER-2 neu positive, and the rest were negative. Five patients were premenopausal and two patients were postmenopausal.

For the seven thermochemotherapy patients with tumors 3.5 cm or greater, based on clinical examination at enrollment, the mean largest perpendicular tumor diameter was 5.68 cm (range 3.5 to 7.5 cm) and the mean tumor area was 27.68 cm2 (range 16 to 45 cm^2) (see **Table 9.4**). Based on ultrasound measurements at enrollment, mean tumor diameter was 2.88 cm (range 2.0 to 4.4 cm) and mean tumor volume was 12.40 cc (range 2.48 to 31.08 cc). All patients completed four cycles of chemotherapy prior to surgery with the exception of Case 1410, in which the tumor was judged (based on ultrasound measurements) to be growing after the first three chemotherapy treatments were administered, and the patient then received a mastectomy. For Case 1410, from the mastectomy specimen the tumor was pathologically 85% necrotic. For the seven patients, mean breast compression during thermotherapy was 5.22 cm, range 3.0 to 6.9 cm. All seven patients (100%) received two treatments of thermotherapy (14 treatments total), but 2 of 14 (14.3%) treatments

Table 9.3 Patient Demographics for Thermochemotherapy-Treated Arm with Tumors 3.5 cm or Greater in Maximum Dimension Based on Clinical Examination

Case	Age (years)/ Menopausal Status	Clinical Tumor Size/ Classification	Tumor Histology	Clinical Nodal Status	Estrogen Receptor Status	Progesterone Receptor Status	HER-2/ neu Status
1102	33, Pre	6.0 cm, T3	IDC	Positive	Negative	Negative	Negative
1403	49, Pre	5.3 cm, T3	IDC	Positive	Negative	Negative	Negative
1406	48, Pre	7.0 cm, T3	IDC	Negative	Negative	Negative	Negative
1409	40, Pre	5.0 cm, T2	IDC	Negative	Negative	Negative	Negative
1410	45, Post	5.0 cm, T2	IDC	Negative	Negative	Negative	Positive
1414	62, Post	4.0 cm, T2	ILC	Negative	Positive	Positive	Negative
1701	26, Pre	7.5 cm, T3	IDC	Negative	Negative	Negative	Negative

IDC, invasive ductal carcinoma ; ILC, invasive lobular carcinoma.

Table 9.4 Subset Results for Tumors 3.5 cm or Greater—Tumor Response and Type of Surgery Following Preoperative Thermotherapy and AC Chemotherapy

Case	Tumor Clinical Classification (size) at Enrollment	Tumor Ultrasound Size (volume) at Enrollment	Peak Tumor Temperature (for two treatments)	CEM Thermal Dose (total for two treatments)	Tumor Size (Shrinkage) by Clinical Exam (area)	Tumor Size (volume) by Ultrasound (Shrinkage)	Type of Surgery (Elligibility based on tumor shrinkage/ Actually Performed)	Tumor Necrosis by H&E Pathology
1102	T3 (6 × 5 cm)	3.9 × 3.9 × 3.9 cm (31.1 cc)	44.6°C	112.4 minutes	0 × 0 cm (100%)	0 × 0 × 0 cm (0 cc) (100%)	BCS/BCS	100%
1403	T3 (5 × 5.3 cm)	2.1 × 1.8 × 2.3 cm (4.56 cc)	46.5°C	233.9 minutes	2.5 × 2.0 cm (81%)	1.76 × 1.0 × 1.01 cm (0.93 cc) (79.6%)	BCS/M	99%
1406	T3 (7 × 4.5 cm)	2.58 × 2.56 × 2.83 cm (9.79 cc)	45.9°C	189.9 minutes	2.0 × 1.75 cm (88.9%)	1.04 × 1.51 × 1.04 cm (0.86 cc) (91.3%)	BCS/BCS	95%
1409	T2 (5 × 5 cm)	2.7 × 2.7 × 2.7 cm (10.31 cc)	46.5°C	193.0 minutes	2.0 × 0.5 cm (96%)	1.23 × 0.97 × 1.29 cm (0.81 cc) (92.2%)	BCS/BCS	95%

(continues)

1410	T2 (5 × 4 cm)	2.02 × 1.63 × 1.44 cm (2.48 cc)	46.1°C	192.3 minutes	4.0 × 4.0 cm (20%)	1.87 × 1.85 × 2.74 cm (4.97 cc) (−99.9%)	M/M	85%
1414	T2 (4 × 3 cm)	2.0 × 2.0 × 2.0 cm (4.16 cc)	46.1°C	224.6 minutes	3.0 × 2.0 cm (62.5%)	1.15 × 1.37 × 1.15 cm (0.95 cc) (77.4%)	BCS/BCS	75%
1701	T3 (7.5 × 6 cm)	4.4 × 2.4 × 4.4 cm (24.35 cc)	45.6°C	108.5 minutes	4.0 × 3.5 cm (68.9%)	2.2 × 2.6 × 1.4 cm (4.2 cc) (82.8%)	BCS/BCS	20%

BCS, breast conservation surgery; CEM, cumulative equivalent minutes; H&E, hematoxylin and eosin; M, mastectomy.

were stopped prior to administering a full thermotherapy dose because of patient discomfort from the thermotherapy treatment.

Thirteen of 14 (92.9%) treatments were administered on the same day as chemotherapy (mean 1.9 hours after chemotherapy, range 1 to 4.1 hours). One thermotherapy treatment was administered 23 hours after chemotherapy. The mean peak tumor temperature achieved for the seven patients was 45.5°C (range 44.6° to 46.5°C), and the mean tumor thermal dose was 190.4 minutes (range 108.5 to 233.9 minutes). For the combination of two thermotherapy treatments, the desired minimum CEM dose of 160 minutes or greater was achieved in 5 of 7 (71.4%) patients.

Prior to surgery, based on clinical examination, the mean tumor diameter was 2.50 cm (range 0 to 4.0 cm) and the mean tumor area was 6.50 cm^2 (range 0 to 16 cm^2). Prior to surgery, based on ultrasound measurements, the mean tumor diameter was 1.49 cm (range 0 to 1.87 cm) and the mean tumor volume was 1.82 cc (range 0 to 4.97 cc). A comparison of tumor dimensions at enrollment with those prior to surgery shows the mean tumor shrinkage based on clinical tumor area was 73.9% (range 20 to 100%), and the mean tumor shrinkage based on ultrasound tumor volume was 60.5% (range−99.9% to 100%). Following thermochemotherapy treatments, based on tumor response in the breast, 6 of 7 (85.7%) patients were eligible for breast conservation. Five of 7 (71.4%) patients actually received breast conservation, and 2 patients received mastectomy. For the 7 patients, mean pathologic tumor necrosis by volume was 81.3% (range 20% to 100%). One of 7 (14.3%) patients had a complete clinical tumor response, and this patient also had a complete pathologic response.

Side effects caused by thermotherapy in the subset group (tumors 3.5 cm or greater) were as follows: fever did not occur for any patients. Erythema (temporary skin redness) was common and occurred in 5 of 7 (71.4%) patients—erythema was more common for patients with larger tumors based on a comparison with the results for the overall population. A skin burn (less than 1.5 cm in size) in the microwave treatment field occurred in 3 of 14 (21.4%) treatments. The patient tolerance of thermotherapy was as follows: patients could tolerate thermotherapy in 13 of 14 (92.9%) treatments, and patients could not tolerate thermotherapy in 1 of 14 (7.1%) treatments.

9.4 DISCUSSION

In this clinical study for patients with T2, T3 tumors, preoperative focused microwave phased array thermotherapy in combination with preoperative AC chemotherapy provided a greater tumor response in terms of tumor shrinkage—median tumor shrinkage based on ultrasound-measured volume was 88.4% in the thermochemotherapy arm (n = 14) compared to 58.8% in the chemotherapy-alone control arm (n = 10)—and was statistically significant ($P = 0.048$). For a subset of patients with large tumors 3.5 cm or greater, 7 of 7 (100%) patients receiving thermochemotherapy exhibited various degrees of tumor necrosis that ranged from 20% to 100%. Based on H&E staining, complete (100%) necrosis of breast cancer was achieved in 1 of 7 (14.3%) patients with large tumors. An increased thermal dose to that used in this study would be required to increase the percentage of patients who achieve a complete pathological tumor response.

Tumor cell kill measured by other pathologic testing such as nicotinamide adenine dinucleotide-diaphorase and immunohistochemistry, as used in other breast tumor ablation studies,[8,9] were not evaluated in this study. The main objective of this study of focused microwave phased array thermotherapy was to determine whether a cumulative thermal dose of 160 equivalent minutes or more could cause tumor shrinkage and tumor ablation without clinically significant toxicity.

The target thermal dose of 160 equivalent minutes was achieved in 5 of 7 (71.4%) patients with tumors 3.5 cm or greater, and the desired peak tumor temperature in the range of 44° to 46°C was achieved in 7 of 7 (100%) patients. Sufficient tumor shrinkage (based on ultrasound measurements) in the breast was achieved such that breast conservation could have been offered to 6 of 7 (85.7%) patients. The actual rate of breast conservation for combining thermotherapy with neoadjuvant AC chemotherapy was 5 of 7 (71.4%) patients. Based on the small study presented here for patients with T2, T3 breast carcinomas, the combined use of thermotherapy and AC chemotherapy appears to be safe and effective.

One advantage of preoperative chemotherapy is the opportunity to observe the chemotherapeutic effect on the primary breast tumor and on any involved axillary nodes, thus allowing an indication of any systemic therapeutic effect the chemotherapy might have on metastatic cancer cells. Because preoperative thermotherapy treatment is localized to the breast, there would be little, if any, effect on the axillary nodes, thus the preoperative chemotherapeutic effect alone can still be observed in the axillary nodes both clinically and pathologically.

From the previous discussions, preoperative focused microwave thermotherapy used in combination with preoperative AC chemotherapy might provide an enhanced therapeutic effect on large carcinomas in the breast, might provide a means for improving the rate of breast conservation, and might increase pathologic tumor cell kill. Because many different drug combinations address patient-specific needs, and many combinations use the common base drug doxorubicin, an alternate study could administer preoperative thermotherapy in combination with doxorubicin and any other standard-of-care drug.

Another AC-based drug combination used in neoadjuvant treatment of invasive breast cancer is fluorouracil, epirubicin, and cyclophosphamide.[10] The AC epirubicin is very similar to doxorubicin in chemical structure. In mice, epidoxorubicin (epirubicin) and paclitaxel (Taxol) cytotoxicity is enhanced at 43°C when the tumors are heated for 60 minutes.[11] A study in sarcoma 180 cells shows enhanced cytotoxicity of doxorubicin and epidoxorubicin when heated at 43°C.[12] Thus, either doxorubicin or epidoxorubicin (as a base chemotherapy agent) potentially could be used equally well in combination with preoperative thermotherapy for enhanced cytotoxicity.

9.5 SUMMARY

Based on the preceding discussions and the results of the study presented in this chapter, preoperative thermotherapy can be administered safely in combination with preoperative AC-based chemotherapy. Ultrasound measurements indicated an improvement in tumor response in the preoperative thermochemotherapy arm compared to the preoperative chemotherapy-alone arm. A future clinical trial for patients with large breast carcinomas, approximately 3.5 cm or greater based on ultrasound measurements, could explore the use of preoperative thermotherapy in combination with preoperative AC-based (doxorubicin or epirubicin) combination chemotherapy versus preoperative AC-based combination chemotherapy alone. This future study could examine the role of thermochemotherapy for increased tumor response and increased use of breast conservation, as well as reduced rate of breast cancer recurrence.

REFERENCES

1. Kaufmann M, Hortobagyi G, Goldhirsch A, et al. Recommendations from an international expert panel on the use of neoadjuvant (primary) systemic treatment of operable breast cancer. An update. *J Clin Oncol.* 2006:24(12): 1940–1949.

2. Fisher B, Brown A, Mamounas E, et al. Effect of preoperative chemotherapy on local-regional disease in women with operable breast cancer: findings from the National Surgical Adjuvant Breast and Bowel Project B-18. *J Clin Oncol.* 1997; 15:2483–2493.

3. Fisher B, Bryant J, Wolmark N, et al. Effect of preoperative chemotherapy in the outcome of women with operable breast cancer. *J Clin Oncol.* 1998;16(8): 2672–2685.

4. Wolmark N, Wang J, Mamounas E, Bryant J, Fisher B. Preoperative chemotherapy in patients with operable breast cancer: nine-year results from National Surgical Adjuvant Breast and Bowel Project B-18. *J Natl Cancer Inst Monogr.* 2001;30:96–102.

5. Vargas HI, Dooley WC, Fenn AJ, et al. Study of preoperative focused microwave phased array thermotherapy in combination with preoperative anthracycline-based chemotherapy of large breast carcinomas. To be submitted to *J Clin Oncol.*

6. Vargas HI, Dooley WC, Gardner RA, Gonzalez KD, Venegas R, Heywang-Kobrunner SH, Fenn AJ. Focused microwave phased array thermotherapy for ablation of early-stage breast cancer: results of thermal dose escalation. *Ann Surg Oncol.* 2004;11(2):139–146.

7. Sapareto SA, Dewey WC. Thermal dose determination in cancer therapy. *Int J Radiat Oncol Biol Phys.* 1984;10:787–800.

8. Gardner RA, Vargas HI, Block JB, Vogel CL, Fenn AJ, Kuehl GV, Doval M. Focused microwave phased array thermotherapy for primary breast cancer. *Ann Surg Oncol.* 2002;9(4):326–332.

9. Huston TL, Simmons RM. Ablative therapies for the treatment of malignant diseases of the breast. *Am J Surg.* 2005;189:694–701.

10. Hamilton A, Hortobagyi G. Chemotherapy: what progress in the last 5 years? *J Clin Oncol.* 2005;23(8):1760–1775.

11. Cividalli A, Livdi E, Ceciarelli F, et al. Hyperthermia and paclitaxel–epirubicin chemotherapy: enhanced cytotoxic effect in a murine mammary adenocarcinoma. *Int J Hyperthermia.* 2000;16(1):61–71.

12. Sakuguchi Y, Maehara Y, Inutsuka S, et al. Laser flow cytometric studies on the intracellular accumulation of anthracyclines when combined with heat. *Cancer Chemother Pharmacol.* 1994;33(5):371–377.

Future Studies

PART

IV

Future Clinical Research Areas for Focused Microwave Breast Thermotherapy

10.1 INTRODUCTION

This book describes the clinical rationale and clinical studies that have been investigated for some of the potential clinical applications of wide-field focused microwave breast thermotherapy. The studies presented here have included preoperative focused microwave thermotherapy for invasive breast cancer (Chapters 6, 7, and 8) as well as preoperative focused microwave thermotherapy in combination with preoperative chemotherapy for treatment of large breast cancer tumors (Chapter 9). Based on the results of these clinical studies in which safety and efficacy have been prospectively explored, future clinical study protocols of diverse applications for treatment of the breast can be considered.[1]

In this chapter, a description of future potential clinical studies for focused microwave thermotherapy for treatment of various types of breast cancer such as early-stage invasive breast cancer (Section 10.2), large breast cancer tumors (Section 10.3), recurrent chest wall breast cancer (Section 10.4), and precancerous ductal carcinoma in situ (DCIS) (Section 10.5) are given. Additional possible clinical research areas for application of focused microwave thermotherapy are also briefly described, including for breast cancer prevention (Section 10.6) and for treating benign breast conditions (Section 10.7).

10.2 PREOPERATIVE THERMOTHERAPY FOR EARLY-STAGE INVASIVE BREAST CANCER IN THE INTACT BREAST

The clinical rationale for treating early-stage invasive breast cancer using preoperative focused microwave thermotherapy to ablate tumor cells was described in Chapter 1—such treatment might improve surgical margins, reduce second incisions, and reduce local recurrence of breast cancer following breast conservation surgery. From the Phase I clinical results presented in Chapter 6, focused microwave heat-alone treatment prior to surgery for small to large breast carcinomas demonstrated safety and breast tumor response in terms of tumor shrinkage and tumor cell kill.[2]

Based on the Phase II preoperative heat-alone thermal dose-escalation results described in Chapter 7 for invasive breast cancers, a predictive minimum thermal dose of 210 equivalent heating minutes for 100% tumor cell kill was established.[3] In Chapter 8, a randomized multicenter study compared focused microwave thermotherapy plus breast conservation surgery to breast conservation surgery alone—tumor cell necrosis was higher in the thermotherapy arm with statistical significance, but higher thermal doses are likely necessary to ensure complete tumor cell kill.[4] In this randomized study, improved margins and fewer second incisions occurred in the focused microwave thermotherapy arm, but statistical significance was not achieved as a result of the small numbers of patients.

As depicted in **Figure 10.1**, future research could investigate larger randomized studies to determine statistically whether preoperative focused microwave thermotherapy improves tumor margins and reduces second incisions compared to current standard-of-care breast conservation, without significant added side effects. Patients could also be followed for 5 to 10 years to determine whether a reduction in local recurrence can be achieved in the preoperative thermotherapy arm compared to current standard-of-care breast conservation.

10.3 PREOPERATIVE THERMOCHEMOTHERAPY FOR LARGE BREAST CANCER TUMORS IN THE INTACT BREAST

Numerous drug combinations have been explored and are being explored for improved neoadjuvant chemotherapy treatment for breast cancer, as described in Chapter 1, Section 1.5. As was shown in Chapter 9, the combined use of neoadjuvant thermotherapy and neoadjuvant anthracycline (AC)–based chemotherapy for T2, T3 tumors can provide increased tumor shrinkage and, for larger tumors

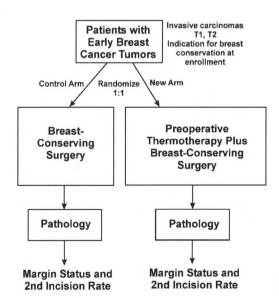

Figure 10.1   Protocol for preoperative thermotherapy with patients with early stage breast cancer vs. standard breast conservation.

3.5 cm or greater, might significantly increase the percentage of patients that can be converted to breast conservation, as well as increase the percentage of patients that achieve a complete pathological tumor response. An increased pathologic tumor response would imply a reduced local recurrence rate for the cancer. An increased pathologic tumor response for decreasing the rate of positive margins could possibly translate into increased survival.[5]

From the previous discussions, preoperative focused microwave thermotherapy used in combination with preoperative AC chemotherapy might provide an enhanced therapeutic effect on large breast cancer tumors in the intact breast,[1] and might provide a means for improving the rate of breast conservation and complete pathologic tumor response, as could be studied in a future clinical trial. In such a clinical trial, thermotherapy in the temperature range of about 44° to 46°C could be administered to large breast cancer tumors (for example, T2 and T3 tumors 3.5 cm or greater) during the first two or three cycles of AC chemotherapy, and the results could be compared against preoperative AC chemotherapy alone in a randomized study. Because many different drug combinations are used preoperatively, and many combinations use the common base drug Adriamycin (doxorubicin), an alternate protocol could administer preoperative thermotherapy in combination with Adriamycin and any other standard-of-care drug.

Another AC-based drug combination for treating breast cancer is fluorouracil, epirubicin, and cyclophosphamide[6] (epirubicin is very similar to doxorubicin in chemical structure, and both drugs (doxorubicin and epirubicin) are enhanced by thermotherapy). Therefore, a future randomized clinical protocol could explore the use of preoperative thermotherapy in combination with preoperative AC-based (doxorubicin or epirubicin) combination chemotherapy versus standard preoperative AC-based combination chemotherapy alone.

Tumors approximately 3.5 cm or larger clinically, with or without skin involvement and without distant metastasis, could be treated with multiple sessions of preoperative focused microwave thermotherapy in combination with preoperative AC-based combination chemotherapy. **Figure 10.2** shows a depiction of a potential protocol that compares preoperative thermochemotherapy with preoperative chemotherapy alone. It is worth pointing out that for large breast carcinomas greater than about 3 to 4 cm clinical examination, mammography, and ultrasound measurements tend to underestimate the pathologic size of tumors.[7] For example, for a clinically measured tumor diameter of 4 cm, the mean pathologic tumor diameter tends to be larger by about 1 cm. Thus, large breast carcinomas tend in many cases to be larger than originally measured prior to the start of treatment, further providing a rationale for a wide-focused microwave thermotherapy treatment field.

10.4 THERMORADIOTHERAPY FOR RECURRENT CHEST WALL BREAST CANCER

Following mastectomy, tumors can recur in the superficial chest wall area (known as *recurrent chest wall cancer*). Recurrent chest wall cancer as well as other superficial cancers are sometimes treated using radiation therapy; however, tumor response rates are low and hyperthermia has been used in combination with radiation therapy to improve response rates.[8-10]

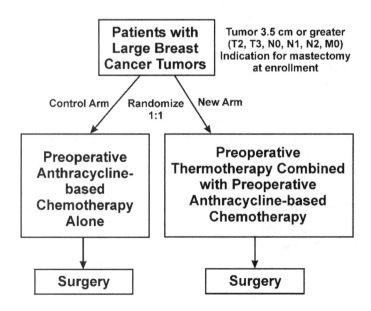

Figure 10.2   Thermochemotherapy vs. chemotherapy alone for patients with large breast cancer tumors in the intact breast.

A recent study by Jones et al[11] has demonstrated a significant improvement in complete response rate for the treatment of superficial tumors (including recurrent chest wall) when hyperthermia is combined with radiation therapy. In that study, between 1994 and 2001, 122 patients at Duke University Medical Center were enrolled with tumors less than 3 cm beneath the skin surface; the complete response rate was 66.1% in the hyperthermia plus radiation arm and 42.3% in the radiation-alone arm. The maximum allowed temperatures in normal tissue and tumor tissue were 43° and 50°C, respectively. In the hyperthermia arm, there were 66% cases of recurrent chest wall cancer, 14% cases of head and neck, 9% cases of melanoma, and 11% other superficial cancers. The hyperthermia dose was in the range of 0.57 to 36.21 thermal equivalent minutes cumulative (relative to 43°C) spread over 10 treatments (2 per week), and skin burns (grade 1 to grade 3) occurred in 46% of patients. Noncoherent spiral array applicators operating at 434 MHz (megahertz) were used to heat the tumors. Although the results with a noncoherent array are encouraging, it might be possible to improve the treatment of recurrent chest wall breast cancer by using an adaptive phased array focused microwave thermotherapy system as has been designed for treatment of the intact breast.[12] In this case, the two microwave applicators would be positioned on the same side of the tissue (chest wall), and the microwave focusing probe would be located 1 to 3 cm deep in the chest wall tissue at the midpoint between the two applicators—the focused microwave thermotherapy treatment might allow deeper penetration of the thermal dose and fewer cold spots between the array applicators compared to a noncoherent array. The treatment protocol would otherwise be the same as the study by Jones et al.[11]

10.5 POSTOPERATIVE THERMOTHERAPY FOR DUCTAL CARCINOMA IN SITU IN THE INTACT BREAST

DCIS, also known as intraductal carcinoma or precancer, in the breast represents a significant therapeutic issue. According to the American Cancer Society, in 2005, for example, there were expected to be 58,490 new cases of in situ breast cancer diagnosed of which an estimated 85% would be DCIS (49,717 new cases of DCIS) and 15% (8,773 new cases) lobular carcinoma in situ (LCIS), in addition to 211,240 new cases of invasive breast cancer.[13] In terms of percentages, in 2005, out of the expected 269,730 cases of new breast cancers diagnosed, 78.3% would be invasive, 18.4% DCIS, and the rest (3.3%) would be LCIS.

A needle biopsy diagnosis of DCIS can underestimate the presence of invasive disease as a result of sampling error, which makes an accurate diagnosis of breast cancer and appropriate treatment difficult. Studies reported by Winchester et al[14] show that 16% to 20% of patients with DCIS diagnosed by needle biopsy were subsequently diagnosed with invasive disease upon surgical excision. *Thus, surgical excision and pathological evaluation of the DCIS-containing breast tissue specimen are currently requirements for DCIS patients to determine an appropriate treatment strategy.*

For example, after an initial diagnosis of DCIS with a subsequent determination of invasive cancer during lumpectomy and pathology, the lymph nodes (particularly the sentinel lymph node[s]) would need to be identified, biopsied, and possibly treated with radiation—stage-appropriate systemic therapy might also be required. *The major goal of any pathologic evaluation of a DCIS patient is to determine the level of risk of subsequent invasion so that proper treatment is offered and possible over- or undertreatment is avoided. Therefore, the addition of any new treatment modality for DCIS must follow the initial surgical excision (lumpectomy) procedure.*

Considering that a cancerous lesion only 0.6 cm in diameter contains on the order of 600 million cancer cells, it is not surprising that residual DCIS cancer cells, or invasive cancer cells as well, can remain in the breast following lumpectomy—some cells are inherently located in a diffuse manner, and some of the cells might also spread during surgery. Whole-breast radiation therapy and a radiation boost administered to the involved region of the breast are commonly administered to kill residual breast DCIS cells. A study of accelerated partial-breast irradiation (twice daily for 5 to 7 days) for DCIS (up to 4.5 cm in maximum dimension based on mammography at enrollment) following surgery has recently been explored by Jeruss et al.[15] Of 158 patients in the study, 37 of 158 (23.42%) had pain caused by radiotherapy, 29 of 158 (18.35%) had subcutaneous tissue changes, 24 of 158 (15.19%) had breast seroma, 18 of 158 (11.39%) had skin contour changes, 17 of 158 (10.76%) had skin erythema, 14 of 158

(8.86%) had skin discoloration, 14 of 158 (8.86%) had late radiation skin changes, and 5 of 158 (3.16%) had breast infection. Radiation dermatitis occurred in 28 of 142 (19.72%) of patients with device-to-skin distance 7 mm or greater and in 9 of 14 (64.29%) of patients with device-to-skin distance 5 to 7 mm. Long-term follow-up of this accelerated partial-breast irradiation approach for DCIS is needed to assess recurrence risk compared to that achieved with whole-breast radiation.

Diagnosis of DCIS is made in about 90% of patients with mammography, and only about 10% of patients will have a palpable mass. The most common mammographic presentation of DCIS is microcalcifications, as described in a review article by Morrow et al[16]— these calcifications tend to be grouped in a cluster, frequently presenting linear or segmental distributions in correlation with their presence in the milk ducts. Typically, no round or oval cluster shapes are found in DCIS, and the extent of DCIS is often underestimated by mammography. Approximately 10% of mammographically detected DCIS cases present without microcalcifications—accurate characterization and visualization of calcifications associated with DCIS typically require magnification of mammographic imaging.

There are several types of DCIS, and they are referred to as *comedo, micropapillary, cribiform, solid,* and *papillary. Comedo* DCIS is the only type likely to present as a palpable mass, and it is also the most likely to be high grade and, as such, *the most likely DCIS type to be associated with concurrent or subsequent invasion.* The histologic features of comedo DCIS are solid growth with central necrosis, often presenting with calcification.

DCIS can be graded based on the Van Nuys system of Silverstein and Lagios. This method relies on differentiating among the three nuclear grades on the basis of four characteristics: (1) size, (2) texture, (3) nucleoli, and (4) the presence or absence of comedo-type necrosis.[17] With these four parameters, tumors can be divided into three graded groups: group 1 (low-grade) tumors with either low- or intermediate-grade nuclei and no necrosis; group 2 (intermediate-grade) tumors with low- or intermediate-grade nuclei and comedo necrosis; and group 3 (high-grade) tumors, which encompasses all tumors with high-grade nuclei regardless of necrosis.

Although tumor grade is a significant prognostic factor for risk of recurrence, other pathologic features can also be of importance. The

Van Nuys grading scheme is part of a prognostic index for DCIS that includes tumor grade, pathologic tumor size, and margin width. In DCIS, however, evaluation of the latter two factors (pathologic tumor size and margin width) can be difficult. Because DCIS does not usually form a grossly visible mass, measurement of the lesion size is almost always done from the pathology slides. It is sometimes difficult to know how to report lesion size when small foci of DCIS are scattered throughout a lumpectomy specimen. Margin width determination is also sometimes very difficult and is an approximation because the sampled pathology slides do not represent a complete depiction of the three-dimensional tumor. Because many recurrences of DCIS probably represent incomplete removal of the DCIS tumor, the issue of margins is critical as described by Silverstein.[18]

Focal DCIS refers to a single isolated spot of DCIS. If the DCIS region is no larger than 4 cm, a lumpectomy can usually be performed. *Multicentric* DCIS means that there are multiple spots or foci with DCIS. *DCIS with extensive intraductal component* means that there are numerous spots with DCIS—mastectomy is usually required in this situation. Local recurrence following total mastectomy is rare, and this is the procedure of choice for DCIS that cannot be adequately treated with breast conservation.

Based on mammographic and pathologic evaluation of the DCIS disease, in some cases breast-conserving surgery can be accomplished with an acceptable cosmetic result. *However, long-term follow-up of DCIS patients treated with complete surgical excision (wide local excision) and radiation therapy shows that, for DCIS characteristics with a higher risk of recurrence, as many as 20% or more experience a local recurrence, with up to 50% of these local recurrences being invasive.*

It is important to observe that DCIS cells can tend to be hypoxic, for which it is known that radiation therapy is less effective as investigated by DeFatta et al.[19] Thus, because of hypoxia, radiation therapy will be limited in its effectiveness against DCIS.

To better understand the impact of local recurrence on survival, consider the following discussion. For DCIS patients who have margin-negative surgery and standard postoperative radiation therapy, at least 80% will achieve long-term local control. With long-term follow-up, approximately 20% of patients experience local recurrences, 10% will have noninvasive recurrence, and 10% will have invasive recurrence. The patients with noninvasive recurrence will achieve virtually 100% local control and cure with mastectomy. The patients with invasive local recurrence will experience a 75% five-year survival rate with mastectomy, that is, 25% will not survive 5 years. Thus, for patients with DCIS managed with breast-conserving treatment, 10% have a noninvasive recurrence and must then have a mastectomy. *The other 10% of patients who have an invasive recurrence must have a mastectomy, and 25% of those patients will die within 5 years. Thus, about 2.5% of patients receiving breast-conserving treatment (lumpectomy and radiation) for DCIS will die within 5 years of local recurrence. Based on the estimated 49,717 DCIS cases in the year 2005, 2.5% of these patients represents 1,243 DCIS patients who will die within 5 years from invasive recurrence.* Given these percentages, most patients will choose a breast-conserving approach; however, these patients will experience significant side effects from the radiation therapy given as part of breast conservation. An alternative treatment to radiation therapy would be desirable in terms of side effects.

For patients with DCIS, local recurrence of breast cancer following excision plus radiation depends on a number of factors as described by Nakamura et al.[20] In Nakamura's article, 260 patients with DCIS at the Van Nuys Breast Center and the USC/Norris Comprehensive Cancer Center from 1979 to 2002 were treated with excision and radiation. A typical radiation therapy whole-breast dose was 5000 cGy (centigray) with a photon boost between 1080 to 1860 cGy in the quadrant of the excised lesion. The risk factors for local recurrence include the DCIS nuclear grade (1 = low grade, 2 = intermediate grade, 3 = high grade), close margin width, tumor size, and subtype. DCIS tumors with intermediate or high grade have higher local recurrences compared to low-grade tumors. DCIS tumors with a surgical close margin width less than 1 cm have a higher local recurrence rate. DCIS tumors that are greater than 1.5 cm have a higher rate of local recurrence. DCIS tumors with a comedo architecture have a higher rate of local recurrence. Cosmetic results of treatment were based on a standard scoring system that evaluated telangiectasia, fibrosis, breast edema, pigmentation, and retraction. In the Nakamura study, the mean tumor size was 1.9 cm at enrollment and the median time to recurrence was 57 months—the rate of local recurrence was 18%, and 46% of the recurrences were invasive (54% were DCIS recurrences).

According to National Comprehensive Cancer Network (NCCN) standard of care (Carlson et al),[21] DCIS patients with widespread disease (two or more involved quadrants) or positive margins at excisional biopsy, with reexcision if desired, receive a total mastectomy without lymph node dissection. If invasive cancer is found pathologically from the excisional biopsy specimen, lymph node management becomes important. The requirement for determining the exact characteristics of the cancer is the reason why DCIS management consists first of accurate diagnostics, and then treatment.

The hypothesis that could be explored in a randomized study protocol for higher risk DCIS patients is that the use of thermotherapy and radiation therapy following lumpectomy can provide increased effectiveness compared to radiotherapy following lumpectomy, with minimal added side effects.[1] In this proposed clinical study, either whole-breast radiation or partial-breast radiation could be considered. Patients could be enrolled in the study if the DCIS tumor has only one involved quadrant or limited volume of the breast, and has one or more of the following characteristics: intermediate- or high-grade tumor, surgical tumor margin less than 1 cm, tumor greater than 1.5 cm in maximum dimension based on pathology, or tumor with comedo architecture. If the addition of thermotherapy to standard breast conservation can reduce the recurrence rate of breast cancer, it might be possible to reduce the number of mastectomies and increase survival if decreased incidence of invasive cancer can be achieved. If, in a future clinical study, thermotherapy can be proved to be as effective as radiation in controlling residual DCIS, thermotherapy might be considered a replacement for radiation therapy because side effects could be reduced.

Approaches for treating DCIS for reducing local recurrence have been investigated in large clinical studies. In the National Surgical Adjuvant Breast and Bowel Project (NSABP) B-17 trial, it was shown that lumpectomy and radiation were more effective than lumpectomy alone for patients with DCIS. In NSABP B-17, 818 women with DCIS and uninvolved margins were randomized to receive wide local excision with or without adjuvant radiotherapy and showed a decrease in local recurrence at 7.5 years follow-up from 27% to 12% with the addition of radiotherapy.[22]

Use of the drug tamoxifen to further reduce breast recurrence after radiation therapy has also been explored. In the NSABP B-24 randomized trial involving 1804 DCIS patients, with 12-year follow-up, treatment with tamoxifen after radiation therapy resulted in a 31% reduction in the average annual incidence rate of ipsilateral breast tumors and a 53% reduction in contralateral breast tumors—the greatest benefit of tamoxifen was in the reduction of invasive breast cancers for both ipsilateral and contralateral events.[23] According to the NCCN guidance,[21,24] there is a uniform consensus based on high-level evidence that tamoxifen treatment can be administered for women with DCIS treated with breast conservation surgery followed by radiation therapy. Toxicities associated with tamoxifen include hot flashes, an increased risk of thromboembolic disease, an increased risk of invasive endometrial cancer in postmenopausal women, and an increased risk of cataracts. An added benefit of tamoxifen is a decrease in bony fractures. Based on the NSABP P-1 trial, tamoxifen was approved for use in the reduction of breast cancer incidence in October 1998. [25]

The hypothesis in this possible randomized study is that the use of breast-conserving surgery followed by focused microwave thermotherapy and radiation therapy can destroy more residual DCIS and other microscopic residual breast carcinomas and provide a local recurrence rate less than a control arm that consists of breast-conserving surgery followed by radiation therapy, and do so with minimal added side effects. Furthermore, if thermotherapy can decrease the rate of recurrence of invasive breast cancer, it might be possible to increase patient survival.

Following surgery, residual DCIS will not present a visible tumor, but rather a surgical cavity possibly with microscopic DCIS at or near the cavity margins. Thermotherapy would be administered following surgery. To treat microscopic DCIS and other carcinomas in the vicinity of the surgical cavity, this randomized study would use an equivalent microwave energy dose as that given in a single treatment for a large group of patients for *lumpectomy plus thermotherapy and radiation therapy, and tamoxifen for eligible patients in the new arm.* In this study, thermotherapy would be administered to residual DCIS approximately 2 to 4 weeks after lumpectomy to allow the breast tissues to heal from surgery before treatment with thermotherapy. Radiation treatment would begin approximately 1 to 2 weeks after thermotherapy. The control arm would use lumpectomy plus radiation therapy and tamoxifen for eligible patients.

Based on the earlier background discussion, the local cancer recurrence rate in the control arm (lumpectomy plus radiation and tamoxifen for eligible patients) would be expected to be 20% at 8 years post treatment. In the new arm, including lumpectomy, thermotherapy, radiation, and tamoxifen for eligible patients, the absolute local cancer recurrence rate could be reduced to 10% post treatment, which would be a significant improvement—such a lower recurrence rate could translate into an improved survival rate.

10.6 BREAST CANCER PREVENTION USING THERMOTHERAPY IN COMBINATION WITH ANTI-ESTROGEN DRUGS

Breast cancer prevention is another therapeutic situation in which thermotherapy could play a role. The current NCCN standard of care for noninvasive or invasive breast cancer prevention is either prophylactic mastectomy (surgical removal of the breasts) or anti-estrogen treatment.[24] Tamoxifen is an anti-estrogen drug that has an affinity for estrogen receptors (ERs), prevents estrogen from binding to breast carcinomas, and prevents tumor growth. Data from the overview of the Early Breast Cancer Trialists' Group indicates that tamoxifen therapy is only effective in those patients that are ER positive.[26]

Raloxifene is another anti-estrogen drug, but currently is inappropriate for breast cancer prevention unless administered within a clinical trial for postmenopausal patients with osteoporosis, as described by Martino et al.[27] Other drugs, such as aromatase inhibitors (for example, anastrozole, trade name Arimidex), reduce the production of estrogen in the breast, as described in a status report by Winer,[28] and these drugs are being evaluated for breast cancer prevention (Cuzick).[29]

In the NSABP P-1 Breast Cancer Prevention Trial[25] performed at 120 investigational sites, 13,175 participants received either tamoxifen (20 mg daily for 5 years) or placebo in a randomized ratio 1:1. Overall, after 69 months follow-up, a 49% reduction in the risk of invasive breast carcinomas was observed in the tamoxifen (trade name

Nolvadex; Zeneca Pharmaceuticals, Wilmington, Delaware) group.[30] For ER-positive patients, the annual rate of breast cancer was 69% less for women in the tamoxifen group versus placebo. For ER negative patients, tamoxifen did not reduce the risk of breast cancer. The NCCN has developed guidelines for Breast Cancer Risk Reduction (in *NCCN Clinical Practice Guidelines in Oncology*, Version 1.2002), including prophylactic mastectomy and tamoxifen therapy.[24]

In NSABP P-1, breast cancer risk assessment was performed for 98,018 patients, and 57,641 patients met the risk eligibility requirements. There were 13,954 patients who met both risk and medical eligibility requirements to participate in the study—13,388 patients were randomly assigned to receive either placebo (6,707 patients) or tamoxifen (6,681 patients).

A total of 368 (2.8%) invasive and noninvasive breast cancers occurred among the 13,175 participants analyzed in NSABP P-1. A total of 6,599 patients received placebo and 6576 patients received tamoxifen in the group of patients that was analyzed in the study. A total of 244 (3.7%) of breast cancers occurred in the placebo group and 124 (1.9%) in the tamoxifen group. There was a highly significant reduction in the incidence of breast cancer as a result of tamoxifen administration; that decrease was observed for both invasive and noninvasive disease. For invasive breast cancer, there was a 49% reduction in the overall risk. There were 175 (2.65%) cases of invasive breast cancer in the placebo group, as compared with 89 (1.35%) in the tamoxifen group ($P < 0.00001$). The cumulative incidence through 69 months was 43.4 per 1000 (4.3%) women and 22.0 per 1000 (2.2%) women in the two groups, respectively. For noninvasive breast cancer, the reduction in risk was 50%; there were 69 cases in women receiving placebo and 35 in those receiving tamoxifen ($P < 0.002$). Through 69 months, the cumulative incidence of noninvasive breast cancer among the placebo group was 15.9 per 1000 (1.59%) women versus 7.7 per 1000 (0.77%) women in the tamoxifen group. The average annual rate of noninvasive breast cancer per 1000 women was 2.68 (0.268%) in the placebo group compared with 1.35 (0.135%) in the tamoxifen group, yielding a relative risk (RR) of 0.50 (95% CI = 0.33 − 0.77). The reduction in noninvasive cancers related to a decrease in the incidence of both DCIS and LCIS. In this study nine deaths were attributed to breast cancer, that is, six in the group that received placebo and three in the tamoxifen group.

In NSABP P-1, rates of invasive breast cancer by selected tumor characteristics were as follows. The annual rate of ER-positive breast cancers was 69% less in women in the tamoxifen group. The annual rates were 5.02 per 1000 (0.502%) women in the placebo group compared with 1.58 per 1000 (0.158%) women in the tamoxifen group (RR = 0.31; 95% CI = 0.22 − 0.45). There was no evidence of a significant difference in the annual rates of tumors presenting as ER-negative (1.20 per 1000 (0.120%) women in the placebo group and 1.46 per 1000 (0.146%) women in the tamoxifen group; RR = 1.22; 95% CI = 0.74 − 2.03).

According to the NSABP P-1 study, tamoxifen administration does not alter the average annual rate of ischemic heart disease; however, a reduction in hip, radius, and spine fractures was observed. The rate of endometrial cancer was increased in the tamoxifen group—this increased risk occurred primarily in women aged 50 years or older.

NSABP P-1 participants who received tamoxifen had a 2.53 times greater risk of developing an invasive endometrial cancer (95% CI = 1.35 − 4.97) than did women who received a placebo, an average annual rate per 1000 participants of 2.30 in the former group and 0.91 in the latter group. The increased risk was predominantly in women 50 years of age or older. The recurrence rate for women aged 49 years or younger was 1.21 (95% CI = 0.41 − 3.60), and it was 4.01 (95% CI = 1.70 − 10.90) in women aged 50 years or older. The increase in incidence after tamoxifen administration was observed early in the follow-up period. Through 66 months of follow-up, the cumulative incidence was 5.4 per 1000 (0.54%) women and 13.0 per 1000 (1.3%) women in the placebo and tamoxifen groups, respectively.

In terms of quality-of-life effects, only hot flashes and vaginal discharge were significant in NSABP P-1.

A novel hypothesis[1] that could be tested is that thermotherapy added to anti-estrogen breast cancer prevention treatment (tamoxifen or other anti-estrogen drugs such as an aromatase inhibitor) versus anti-estrogen drugs alone can reduce the risk of invasive breast carcinomas by increasing the amount of blockage of estrogen to the ERs of breast carcinomas—without added side effects. The amount of increased blockage of estrogen could be achieved by damaging or modifying high-water-content/high-ion-content ERs with focused microwaves. In addition, thermotherapy could kill microscopic breast carcinoma cells directly with heat either by necrosis or apoptosis, which would be efficacious for both ER-positive and ER-negative patients. Patients in the thermotherapy and tamoxifen arm would receive the standard dose of tamoxifen (20 mg per day for 5 years) and thermotherapy at 2.5-year intervals during the same 5-year period. Because patients in this clinical trial would not have an identifiable lesion, the target region could simply be the upper portion (inner and outer quadrants) of the breast where a majority of all breast cancers occur—45% upper outer quadrant, 15% upper inner quadrant, 25% nipple region, 10% lower outer quadrant, and 5% lower inner quadrant.[31] For thermotherapy treatment targeting the upper portion of the breast, breast compression could be in the cranial-caudal position and the E-field focusing probe could be positioned toward the cranial side of the breast. However, for the compressed breast treatment with opposed microwave applicators where the microwaves penetrate through the breast, a majority of the breast is treated with the exception of the nipple. Skin temperature sensors would be monitored and the microwave power of the two channels would be adjusted to keep skin temperatures below about 41°C during the thermotherapy treatment so that the skin will not burn or blister. Therefore, a microwave energy dose could be administered to the breast in each of multiple (a few) treatments spaced at, say, approximately 2.5-year intervals during the period of administration of tamoxifen. The control group for this clinical trial would include patients receiving only tamoxifen treatment (20 mg per day) for 5 years.

As mentioned earlier, a total of 368 (2.8%) invasive and noninvasive breast cancers occurred among the 13,175 participants analyzed in NSABP P-1. In a future clinical study, a total of approximately 2500 patients in the control arm could receive anti-estrogen drugs alone and 2500 patients in the new arm could receive anti-estrogen drugs and thermotherapy. If tamoxifen was the anti-estrogen drug used in the study, using round numbers, a total of 50 (2%) breast cancers would be expected to develop in the tamoxifen-alone control arm. If thermotherapy and tamoxifen in combination are effective, then the rate of the occurrence of breast cancer could drop to, say, 1.0% (or 25 patients), which would be a statistically significant result (80% power to detect a difference between the two arms at a significance level of 0.05). This hypothesized breast cancer prevention protocol could be a long-term goal for application of focused microwave phased array thermotherapy.

10.7 THERMOTHERAPY TREATMENT OF BENIGN BREAST CONDITIONS

Benign (nonmalignant) breast conditions are the most common nonmalignant breast disorder of women in which *breast pain is the major symptom*. Other names for benign breast conditions are "benign breast lesions," "benign breast disease," "mammary dysplasia," "fibrocystic breast disease," "fibrocystic breast conditions," "mastalgia," and "chronic cystic mastitis." The commonly used expression "benign breast conditions" covers a broad range of benign conditions from painful breasts with solid lumpy patches to cysts (lumps filled with fluid). A classification guide (Columbia Classification) for benign breast conditions, as described by Haagensen et al,[32] is as follows:

a. Microscopic features (blunt ducts, microcysts less than 3 mm in diameter, and apocrine epithelium) normally seen in the breast. They do not form a palpable tumor and do not predispose to subsequent carcinoma.

b. Microscopic lesions (adenosis, papillomatosis) frequently seen in the breasts of women, but not often enough to be regarded as normal components. They do not form a palpable tumor (except for extensive adenosis) and do not predispose to subsequent carcinoma.

c. Clinically evident lesions (fibrous disease, fibroadenoma, solitary intraductal papilloma in a subareolar terminal duct), which often form a palpable tumor, but do not predispose to subsequent breast carcinoma.

d. Microscopic or clinically evident lesions ("benign" atypical ductal hyperplasia [BADH] and gross cysts 3 mm or more in diameter), which might or might not form a palpable tumor but do predispose to subsequent carcinoma. The relative risk of breast cancer from these lesions is as follows: gross cysts, 1.3% and 2.7% without and with first-degree family history, respectively; BADH, 4.4% and 8.9% without and with first-degree family history, respectively.[33] It should be noted that the stage following BDAH is DCIS. It could be potentially important to ablate BDAH cells before they become DCIS.

    e. Clinically evident breast lesions (multiple intraductal papilloma and gross cysts), which form a palpable tumor and do predispose to carcinomas.

Benign fibroadenomas are a particularly common benign breast tumor. Approximately 500,000 new cases of breast fibroadenoma are detected annually in the United States. Current treatment for fibroadenoma consists of surgical excision, or more recently office-based ultrasound-guided cryoablation is being explored, as described by Kauffman et al.[34] Cryoablation has been used to treat benign fibroadenomas up to 4 cm in diameter. Focused microwave thermotherapy is an approach that could be used to treat single or multiple fibroadenomas for sizes or distributions up to about 8 to 10 cm in maximum dimension.

Benign breast conditions are common among women of childbearing years, and many *women suffer from moderate to severe pain from benign breast conditions*. Pain killers (analgesics such as naproxen sodium) and a growth hormone inhibitor (danazol) are currently the only Food and Drug Administration (FDA)–approved treatments for pain from benign breast conditions. Analgesics provide only temporary relief from pain and do not treat the disease. The FDA-approved hormone inhibitor danazol, taken 100–200 mg twice daily orally for breast pain, has numerous side effects.[35] Breast pain progressively increases as a result of increasing amounts of benign breast condition tissue as the patient ages. Other treatments explored in the United Kingdom such as bromocriptine, tamoxifen, and gamolenic acid (primrose oil) for pain associated with benign breast conditions have demonstrated a benefit, but are not FDA approved. Benign breast condition tissue can cause monthly cyclic pain and tenderness. The symptoms often occur typically one week before the menstrual cycle begins (day 1 of the menstrual cycle is designated as that day on which menstrual flow begins) and often subside about one week later.

Benign breast lesions such as cysts are rarely malignant, but in a very few cases (about 1%), a small carcinoma might grow inside the cyst without spreading into the surrounding breast tissue. Cysts are fluid-filled sacs, very much like a large blister.

As described in Chapter 2, Section 2.4, benign lesions such as cysts, fibroadenomas, fibrosis, fibroadrosis, and epitheliosis (also known as papillomatosis) are high water and/or high ion content and should be readily heated by microwave energy compared to the heating of surrounding normal healthy breast tissue. The hypothesis[1] that could be explored in a future study is whether the use of focused microwave thermotherapy and analgesics can decrease the size of and destroy benign breast lesions and reduce breast pain compared to a control arm using pain killers (analgesics) only. Another hypothesis[1,36] that could be considered is whether the use of focused microwave thermotherapy alone can destroy benign breast lesions such as fibroadenomas or cysts—while heating these lesions, any undetected breast carcinoma cells in the field of the microwave applicators might be heated and destroyed. To prove either of these hypotheses, large randomized clinical studies would be required.

10.8 SUMMARY

This chapter has described a number of possible clinical studies that could be considered in the future for treating the intact breast using adaptive phased array focused microwave thermotherapy. Preoperative focused microwave thermotherapy could be further studied as a heat-alone treatment prior to surgery to reduce the incidence of positive surgical margins, reduce breast surgery, and reduce local recurrence rate. Preoperative focused microwave thermotherapy used in combination with preoperative chemotherapy could be further researched to provide increased tumor shrinkage and improve the rate of breast conservation for large breast cancer tumors or increase the rate of complete pathologic response, and possibly improve survival. Focused microwave thermotherapy in combination with radiation therapy could be explored for patients with recurrent chest wall breast cancer. Postoperative thermotherapy could be explored to treat precancerous DCIS and reduce the recurrence rate of invasive breast cancer, which could improve survival. Use of thermotherapy in combination with anti-estrogen drugs could be explored to prevent breast cancer by damaging ERs and killing microscopic breast cancer cells. Use of thermotherapy in combination with analgesics could be explored to relieve breast pain for benign breast conditions by targeting and destroying high-water-/high-ion-content lesions.

It has been recently reported that cancer stem cells might be a significant source for generating cancerous tumors. Cancer stem cells are reported to be resistant in many cases to chemotherapy and can persist after surgery and lead to recurrence as discussed by Perryman and

Sylvester.[37] Out of the roughly 1 billion cancer cells that can exist in a 1-cm tumor, there are speculated to be on the order of 1000 cancer stem cells (one stem cell per million cells)—if focused microwave thermotherapy can target and kill these aggressive stem cells in tumors, perhaps it is possible to reduce or prevent further tumor growth and spread of malignant cells. Whether cancer stem cells are high water and high ion content and subject to rapid heating and cell death by focused microwave thermotherapy remain to be investigated.

Although not described here, other clinical applications for focused microwave thermotherapy are possible. In contrast with photodynamic therapy,[38] which uses laser light to energize drugs, deep heating with an adaptive phased array focused microwave thermotherapy system can be used to activate thermosensitive liposomes to concentrate a drug into a tumor region and increase the effectiveness of the drug. The word *thermodynamics* refers to the physics of the relationship between heat and other forms of energy.[39] Thus, the treatment technique of drug delivery and activation by heat can be referred to as a thermodynamic therapy.[40] Focused microwave thermotherapy using adaptive phased arrays has potential application, in combination with radiation therapy, chemotherapy, or targeted drug delivery with thermosensitive liposomes (thermodynamic therapy), in the treatment of cancers such as primary breast cancer; recurrent breast cancer; and head and neck, liver, prostate, colon, rectum, cervical, ovarian, and lung cancers.[40] Wide-field focused microwave adaptive phased array thermotherapy for treatment of various types of breast cancers and a wide variety of cancers other than in the breast can be the subject of a number of future clinical studies.

REFERENCES

1. Fenn AJ, Mon J. Thermotherapy method for treatment and prevention of breast cancer and cancer in other organs. US Patent Number 6,690,976. February 10, 2004.

2. Gardner RA, Vargas HI, Block JB, Vogel CL, Fenn AJ, Kuehl GV, Doval M. Focused microwave phased array thermotherapy for primary breast cancer. *Ann Surg Oncol.* 2002;9(4):326–332.

3. Vargas HI, Dooley WC, Gardner RA, Gonzalez KD, Venegas R, Heywang-Kobrunner SH, Fenn AJ. Focused microwave phased array thermotherapy for ablation of early-stage breast cancer: results of thermal dose escalation. *Ann Surg Oncol.* 2004;11(2):139–146.

4. Dooley WC, Vargas HI, Fenn, AJ, et al. Randomized study of preoperative focused microwave phased array thermotherapy for early-stage invasive breast cancer. To be submitted to *Ann of Surg Oncol.*

5. Rapiti E, Verkooijen HM, Vlastos G, et al. Complete excision of primary breast tumor improves survival of patients with metastatic breast cancer at diagnosis. *J Clin Oncol.* 2006;24(18):2743–2749.

6. Kaufmann M, Hortobagyi G, Goldhirsh A, et al. Recommendations from an international expert panel on the use of neoadjuvant (primary) systemic treatment of operable breast cancer. An update. *J Clin Oncol.* 2006:24(12):1940–1949.

7. Heusinger K, Lohberg C, Lux MP, et al. Assessment of breast tumor size depends on method, histopathology and tumor size itself. *Breast Cancer Res Treat.* November 2005;94(1):17–23.

8. Vernon CC, Hand JW, Field SB et al. Radiotherapy with or without hyperthermia in the treatment of superficial localized breast cancer: results from five randomized controlled trials. *Int J Rad Oncol Biol Phys.* 1996;35:731–744.

9. Overgaard J, Gonzalez Gonzalez D, Hulshof MC, et al. Randomized trial of hyperthermia as an adjuvant to radiotherapy for metastatic malignant melanoma. *Lancet.* 1995;345:540–543.

10. Valdagni R, Amichetti, M. Report of long-term follow-up in a randomized trial comparing radiation therapy and radiation therapy plus hyperthermia to metastatic lymph nodes in stage IV head and neck patients. *Int J Rad Oncol Biol Phys.* 1993;28:163–169.

11. Jones EL, Oleson JR, Prosnitz LR, et al. Randomized trial of hyperthermia and radiation for superficial tumors. *J Clin Oncol.* May 1, 2005;23(13):3079–3085.

12. Fenn AJ, Wolf GL, Fogle RM. An adaptive phased array for targeted heating of deep tumours in intact breast: animal study results. *Int J Hyperthermia.* 1999;15(6):45–61.

13. American Cancer Society. *Cancer Facts & Figures 2005*. Atlanta, Ga: American Cancer Society; 2005.

14. Winchester DP, Jeske JM, Goldschmidt RA. The diagnosis and management of ductal carcinoma in-situ of the breast. *CA Cancer J Clin*. 2000;50:184–200.

15. Jeruss JS, Vicini FA, Beitsch PD, et al. Initial outcomes for patients treated on the American Society of Breast Surgeons MammoSite clinical trial for ductal carcinoma-in-situ of the breast. *Ann Surg Oncol*. 2006;13(7):967–976.

16. Morrow M, Strom EA, Bassett LW, et al. Standard for the management of ductal carcinoma in situ of the breast (DCIS). *CA Cancer J Clin*. September/October 2002;52(5):256–276.

17. Silverstein MJ, Lagios MD, Craig PH, et al. A prognostic index for ductal carcinoma in situ of the breast. *Cancer*. 1996;77:2267–2274.

18. Silverstein MJ, Lagios MD, Goshen S, et al. The influence of margin width on local control of ductal carcinoma in situ of the breast. *N Engl J Med*. 1999;340:1455–1461.

19. DeFatta RJ, Turbat-Herrera EA, Li BDL, et al. Elevated expression of eIF4E in confined early breast cancer lesions: possible role of hypoxia. *Int J Cancer*. 1999;80:516–522.

20. Nakamura SK, Woo C, Silberman H, et al. Breast-conserving therapy for ductal carcinoma in situ: a 20-year experience with excision plus radiation. *Am J Surg*. 2002;(184):403–409.

21. Carlson RW, Anderson BO, Bensinger W, et al. The NCCN Breast Cancer Clinical Guidelines in Oncology. *J Natl Compr Cancer Network*. 2003;1:148–188.

22. Fisher B, Dignam J, Wolmark N, et al. Lumpectomy and radiation therapy for the treatment of intraductal breast cancer: findings from National Surgical Adjuvant Breast and Bowel Project B-17. *J Clin Oncol*. 1998;16:441–452.

23. Fisher B, Land S, Mamounas E, et al. Prevention of invasive breast cancer in women with ductal carcinoma in situ, an update of the National Surgical Adjuvant Breast and Bowel Project experience. *Semin Oncol*. 2001;28:400–418.

24. Carlson TW, Bevers TB, Blackwell KL, et al. The NCCN Breast Cancer Risk Reduction Clinical Guidelines in Oncology. *J Natl Compr Cancer Network*. 2003;1:280–296.

25. Fisher, B, Costantino JP, Wickerham DL, et al. Tamoxifen for prevention of breast cancer: report of the National Surgical Adjuvant Breast and Bowel Project P-1 Study. *J Natl Cancer Inst*. 1998;90:1371–1388.

26. Early Breast Cancer Trialists' Collaborative Group. Tamoxifen for early breast cancer: an overview of the randomised trials. *Lancet*. 1998;351:1451–1467.

27. Martino S, Cauley JA, Barrett-Connor E, et al. Incidence of invasive breast cancer following 8 years of raloxifene therapy in postmenopausal women with osteoporosis: results from the Continuing Outcomes Relevant to Evista (CORE) trial. *Proc Am Soc Clin Oncol.* 2004;23:97. Abstract 1000.

28. Winer EP. American Society of Clinical Oncology Technology Assessment on the use of aromatase inhibitors as adjuvant therapy for postmenopausal women with hormone receptor–positive breast cancer: status report 2004. *J Clin Oncol.* 2005;23(3):619–629.

29. Cuzick J. Aromatase inhibitors for breast cancer prevention. *J Clin Oncol.* 2005;23(8):1636–1643.

30. Morrow M, Jordan VC. Tamoxifen for the prevention of breast cancer in the high-risk woman. *Ann Surg Oncol.* 2000;7(1):67–71.

31. National Council on Radiation Protection and Measurements. *Mammography— A User's Guide.* Bethesda, Md: National Council on Radiation Protection and Measurements; 1987:7. NCRP Report No. 85.

32. Haagensen CD, Bodian C, Haagensen DE. *Breast Carcinoma, Risk and Detection.* Philadelphia, Pa: WB Saunders; 1981.

33. Love S. *Dr. Susan Love's Breast Book.* 4th ed. Cambridge, MA: DeCapo Press; 2005:207.

34. Kauffman CS, Bachman B, Littrup PJ, et al. Office-based ultrasound-guided cryoablation of breast fibroadenomas. *Am J Surg.* 2002;184:394–400.

35. Love S. *Dr. Susan Love's Breast Book.* 4th ed. Cambridge, MA: DeCapo Press; 2005:59–66.

36. Fenn AJ, Mon J. Method for heating ductal and glandular carcinomas and other breast lesions to perform thermal downsizing and a thermal lumpectomy. US Patent Number 6,470,217. October 22, 2002.

37. Perryman SV, Sylvester KG. Repair and regeneration: opportunities for carcinogenesis from tissue stem cells. *J Cellular Molecular Medicine.* 2006;10(2):292–308.

38. Shum P, Kim JM, Thompson DH. Phototriggering of liposomal drug delivery systems. *Adv Drug Delivery Rev.* 2001;53:273–284.

39. Sommerfeld A. *Thermodynamics and Statistical Mechanics: Lectures on Theoretical Physics.* In: Bopp F, Meixner J, Kestin J, eds. New York, NY: Academic Press; 1961; V.

40. Fenn AJ. Thermodynamic adaptive phased array system for activating thermosensitive liposomes in targeted drug delivery. US Patent Number 5,810,888. September 22, 1998.

Index